SEXUAL LIFE
A CLINICIAN'S GUIDE

CRITICAL ISSUES IN PSYCHIATRY
An Educational Series for Residents and Clinicians

Series Editor: Sherwyn M. Woods, M.D., Ph.D.
University of Southern California School of Medicine
Los Angeles, California

Recent volumes in the series:

CASE STUDIES IN INSOMNIA
Edited by Peter J. Hauri, Ph.D.

CHILD AND ADULT DEVELOPMENT: A Psychoanalytic Introduction
for Clinicians
Calvin A. Colarusso, M.D.

CLINICAL DISORDERS OF MEMORY
Aman U. Khan, M.D.

CONTEMPORARY PERSPECTIVES ON PSYCHOTHERAPY WITH LESBIANS
AND GAY MEN
Edited by Terry S. Stein, M.D., and Carol J. Cohen, M.D.

DECIPHERING MOTIVATION IN PSYCHOTHERAPY
David M. Allen, M.D.

DRUG AND ALCOHOL ABUSE: A Clinical Guide to Diagnosis and Treatment,
Third Edition
Marc A. Schuckit, M.D.

ETHNIC PSYCHIATRY
Edited by Charles B. Wilkinson, M.D.

EVALUATION OF THE PSYCHIATRIC PATIENT: A Primer
Seymour L. Halleck, M.D.

THE FREEDOM OF THE SELF: The Bio-Existential Therapy
of Character Problems
Eugene M. Abroms, M.D.

HANDBOOK OF BEHAVIOR THERAPY IN THE PSYCHIATRIC SETTING
Edited by Alan S. Bellack, Ph.D., and Michel Hersen, Ph.D.

NEUROPSYCHIATRIC FEATURES OF MENTAL DISORDERS
James W. Jefferson, M.D., and John R. Marshall, M.D.

RESEARCH IN PSYCHIATRY: Issues, Strategies, and Methods
Edited by L. K. George Hsu, M.D., and Michel Hersen, Ph.D.

SEXUAL LIFE: A Clinician's Guide
Stephen B. Levine, M.D.

STATES OF MIND: Configurational Analysis of Individual Psychology,
Second Edition
Mardi J. Horowitz, M.D.

A Continuation Order Plan is available for this series. A continuation order will bring
delivery of each new volume immediately upon publication. Volumes are billed only upon
actual shipment. For further information please contact the publisher.

SEXUAL LIFE
A CLINICIAN'S GUIDE

Stephen B. Levine, M.D.

Center for Human Sexuality
Department of Psychiatry
University Hospitals of Cleveland
Case Western Reserve University School of Medicine
Cleveland, Ohio

PLENUM PRESS • **NEW YORK AND LONDON**

Library of Congress Cataloging-in-Publication Data

Levine, Stephen B., 1942-
    Sexual life : a clinician's guide / Stephen B. Levine.
        p.   cm. -- (Critical issues in psychiatry)
    Includes bibliographical references and index.
    ISBN 0-306-44287-6
    1. Psychosexual disorders. 2. Sex therapy. 3. Sex.   I. Title.
II. Series.
RC566.L47 1992
616.8'583--dc20   92-28033
                                                              CIP

ISBN 0-306-44287-6

© 1992 Plenum Press, New York
A Division of Plenum Publishing Corporation
233 Spring Street, New York, N. Y. 10013

Printed in the United States of America

To Lillian, my wife

Foreword

There has been great progress in recent years in our understanding of human sexuality, both normal and disordered. Few health professionals, and especially mental health professionals, can spend a day with patients without encountering some form of suffering related to sexuality. Problems vary enormously with respect to nature, severity, and treatment approach. This book addresses the entire range, and does so with great effectiveness.

Effective clinical management requires the truly biopsychosocial understanding and treatment strategies so clearly presented by Dr. Levine. His approach to patients is simultaneously sensitive, practical, sophisticated, and comprehensive. His conceptualization of diagnosis and treatment integrates behavioral, cognitive, and psychodynamic thinking, and always does so with an eye to relevant biological dimensions.

I am especially pleased to welcome this book to the series, because it will have an important place in the education of psychiatric residents and other mental health professionals. The depth and quality of the presentation, however, make it equally rewarding reading for the most experienced of clinicians.

SHERWYN M. WOODS, M.D., PH.D.
Series Editor

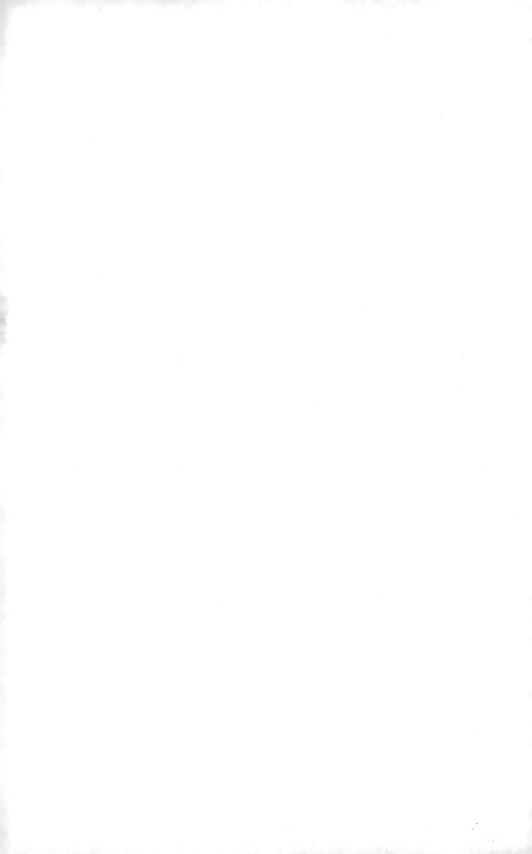

Preface

It has been almost two decades since I began listening to single and married people talk about their sexual concerns. This privileged position has helped me to better understand my personal development and my role as a therapist and to realize that I have a definable perspective on sexual life.

I remain enamored of the opportunities to learn and to help that exist within the roles of clinician and teacher. It never ceases to be a delight to be of assistance to another person or a couple, or to open the door to an understanding of the sexual universe for a student. Always hovering near these pleasures, however, is the awareness of what is not understood. I have come to view genuine expertise as that which exists when a person is acutely aware of the limits of knowledge. I greatly admire those clinicians and behavioral scientists, many of whom are referenced in this book, whose scholarship and research have pushed our understanding of sexuality a notch or two further or who have cogently articulated the previously inapparent limits of our knowledge.

Over the years, I have been encouraged by the interest of mental health trainees in my emerging perspectives. I became sufficiently emboldened to write this book, in part, because of the pleasure of watching these trainees make sense of their patients' sexual concerns using these perspectives.

Sexual Life has arisen from the many stimulating interactions with individuals and couples in therapy, trainees in individual supervision, and groups in the small conferences held three times a week at the Center for Human Sexuality (part of the Department of Psychiatry). I owe an enormous debt of gratitude to the many persons in each of these categories. It is inconceivable to me that this book could have been written without them.

Those who are aware of what the Center for Human Sexuality is, and what it aspires to be, know that none of its therapy, education, or research could have been conducted without the devoted efforts of Stanley Althof,

Ph.D., and Candace Risen, L.I.S.W., who have been my teammates since the time when all of us considered ourselves young. To these two talented, wonderful people, in particular, and to the many Fellows in Sexuality who have spent one or two years helping us do our work, I offer my affection and lasting gratitude.

Contents

Chapter 7

The Sexual Equilibrium 79

Chapter 8

Helping Men to Control Ejaculation 90

Chapter 9

Helping Women to Become Orgasmic 107

CHAPTER 1

What Is Sexuality?

Sexuality is an everpresent, ever-evolving, multifaceted possession of every human being. Encased in five layers of privacy, it contains the subtle dramas of our development.

THE MEANING OF "SEXUALITY"

The word *sexuality* has no precise definition. This fact enables the term to be employed by any individual with unknowing impunity in speech and print. Listeners or readers rarely ask the reasonable questions, "What are you talking about? What do you mean by sexuality?" Everyone either grasps the definition from contextual cues, assigns it a private meaning, or simply pretends to understand.

Within the health care professions, the term *sexuality* refers to personal characteristics involving anatomy, reproduction, identity, genital responses, or physical disease. For example, the phrase "his sexuality is a problem" might describe a male's physical or psychological features, such as his malformed penis, infertility, attraction to children, premature ejaculation, or HIV (human immunosuppressive virus) infection.

Sexuality is relevant as well to the world of marketing, where powerful interpersonal attraction and excitement are important. Ever attuned to selling, the commercial world distorts and exploits the superficial interpersonal aspects of sexuality to achieve its material goals.

Sexuality, however, is neither a disease nor a commodity. It is an everpresent, ever-evolving, multifaceted resource of every human being. It has far more to do with health and the unfolding of our lives than with illness. Health care professionals have a practical but narrow slant on the subject. Generally, we are interested in sexuality as it relates to physical or mental problems. Sexuality is part of every human being, but disease afflicts only a small portion of a population at any time.

Sexuality begins in the biology of genes and chromosomes that direct the creation and evolution of anatomic structures and physiological pro-

1

cesses. These, in turn, partially shape many psychological dimensions of sexuality. The details of the biologic development of sexuality are still largely mysterious. Far less mysterious are the forces that assault our sexuality once our adult sexual dimensions are formed. Medical doctors tend to know about the organic assaults on sexuality, whereas mental health professionals concentrate on the psychological and social assaults. In order to understand more fully the biological, psychological, and social influences on sexuality, mental health clinicians need to know how sexuality relates to health and happiness, as well as to illness and distress. Before delineating eight perspectives on the meanings of sexuality to clinicians, I want to clarify the role of mental health professionals.

THE DEVELOPMENT OF CLINICIANS

The mental health professions offer their members the familiar activities of patient care, administration, education, and research. Most individuals are attracted to the field by images of patient care, and have their first clinical experiences after a relatively brief conceptual introduction to mental illness. What happens during these early clinical encounters often determines whether mental health professionals will sustain their interest in direct care and become competent clinicians or gravitate to one or more of the other legitimate roles.

Clinicians are mental health professionals who enjoy trying to help emotionally distressed people. Rather than feeling frightened, helpless, or bored by patients' distress, clinicians are often engrossed by it. Clinicians feel privileged to listen to stories about events and people that few persons hear. These stories, usually told with a genuineness that provides a unique perspective, quickly expand the life experiences of the clinician.

As clinicians, we soon learn to be engaged emotionally and intellectually while listening. We react within our private selves to much of what we hear, and use these feelings and memories to help us to synthesize the person's problem. Countless repetitions of the active clinical processes of listening, reacting, and synthesizing eventually enable us to view simultaneously both the unique and similar characteristics of our patients. Our appreciation of their uniqueness sustains our relationship to them; our recognition of the similarity of their distress to that of other patients permits accurate diagnosis and traditional therapy planning. This dual appreciation of our patients gradually creates the legitimacy of our identities as clinicians.[1] It also helps us to realize how different we clinicians are from the many nonprofessionals who are capable of high quality relationships and from other mental health professionals whose activities do not involve patient care.

As our clinical experiences with the distressed accumulate, we learn to articulate some of the causes of our patients' anguish. This is a vital step in the development of a clinician because being therapeutic often depends on the clinician's ability to remove the mystery of the origin and maintenance of the person's misery. This new, hard-won ability generates deep satisfaction because competence in this role is widely understood to mean the ability to relieve emotional distress.

If clinicians devote themselves to the art of being therapeutic for several decades, they experience a subtle, enriching evolution of their perspective on their work. The types of problems they choose to deal with, however, do not essentially modify the challenges, social expectations, or rewards of clinicians. Clinicians can expect a similar professional maturation whether they see patients with mood, anxiety, thought, or sexual disorders.

"WHAT IS SEXUALITY?" EIGHT ANSWERS

Although not one of these answers alone is sufficient to convey the complexity of sexuality, taken together, they introduce us to the subject.

1. Sexuality is an energy-driven psychological *vehicle* for pleasure, self-discovery, attachment, and self-esteem. The source of this energy, although unknown, is whatever provides the momentum for psychological development throughout life.
2. Sexuality is a private experience of *identity* contributed to by our sense of our anatomy, physiology, gender identity, orientation, and intention. There are other identities besides sexual, but none are as consistently central to mental functioning from person to person.
3. Sexuality is our *physiological capacity* for desire, arousal, and orgasm and its exquisite responsiveness to social and psychological forces. Sexual physiological capacity has its own biology and evolution during the life cycle.
4. Sexuality is a *resource* that can be well managed into personal contentment, good mental health, and self and partner love or poorly managed into despair, premature or unvalued pregnancy, venereal disease, and death.
5. Sexuality is our repertoire of *intimate physical behaviors* with partners and the many meanings that we, our partners, and our culture give to these interactions.
6. Sexuality is an *emotional response system* that orients us to ourselves and to other people. It is a type of inner voice, a running dialogue within our privacy, that sheds light on our psychological selves at every stage of life. This voice speaks to us of our current needs for

attachment to others and our comfort in being with a particular partner. It is a voice of truth, often an unsociable, unkind voice, which is ignored at great peril. The voice alerts us to the state of our attitudes about our partners and others in our lives.

7. Sexuality is a *repair mechanism* with the power to fix our troubled sense of self by cutting loose our painful pasts and allowing us to experience our bodies and our selves as good and lovable, even though in younger years we may have experienced them with uncertainty or guilt.

8. Sexuality is a *vantage point* from which to study the psychology of individuals and couples—particularly how their intimate relationships form, evolve, and dissolve. Sexuality is a window to the drama of our inner lives, particularly our struggle to love. This struggle, until recently, has been largely ignored by the mental health professions.[2,3]

These inexact, overlapping definitions constitute opportunities for mental health professionals to learn about life processes, not just problems. The study of sexuality is germane to almost every type of problem clinicians take care of; few clinical problems are without sexual implications.

SEXUALITY AND THE NEED FOR PRIVACY

Most of our sexuality is enveloped in a protective shield of privacy. This shield is composed of mutually reinforcing layers that keep other people from knowing about our sexual selves. These layers are so consistently impenetrable that privacy is accepted as a fundamental psychological requirement of sexual expression beyond early childhood. The role of clinician necessitates that these layers be temporarily, carefully, and respectfully parted.

The Distinction between Secrecy and Privacy

It is important to grasp the distinction between *privacy* and *secrecy* in order to understand how this protective shield operates. A fact is considered a secret when a person does not want another person to know of its existence. Masturbation is viewed as a secret by many young adolescents, for instance. If a person with a secret is confronted, lies, denials, illogic, or irrational behaviors quickly arise to obscure the fact and maintain the secret.

MOTHER (upon walking into the teenager's bedroom unannounced): "Are you masturbating?"
TEENAGER: "No. I was fixing my sheets. (Screaming) Get out of here!"

A fact that is acknowledged to exist although the details are socially off-limits is considered to be a privacy. For instance, respectful parents consider their teenager's masturbation a private matter. Here is a more complicated example:

"Daddy, do you and mommy have intercourse?"
"Yes, dear, we do." (The fact of parental intercourse is no cause for secrecy.)
"Daddy, did you and mommy have intercourse last night?"
"That's none of your business, dear." (A child's curiosity is no cause to abandon the privacy of the marital sexual relationship.)

A child, curious to know about the universe, inevitably has questions about sexuality. Many children grow up never having been able to ask their questions. If they have asked them, they often have not been satisfactorily answered because their parents and their culture could not make the distinctions between secrecy and privacy. It is no secret that children, adolescents, and adults have sexual feelings, behaviors, curiosities, and inhibitions. The facts about this can be presented without embarrassment as long as the boundaries of privacy are respected. Clinicians have to know the facts and be willing to discuss them, all the while respecting the important boundaries of privacy. This is often easier said than done because clinicians' own internal responses to hearing about the sexuality of others may make them unwilling to continue to address the topic.

Clinicians sometimes respond with mild arousal when listening to sexual details of another person's life. If this is misunderstood by the young clinician and labeled as an unethical reaction, sexual topics during psychotherapy may be subsequently avoided.* In addition, what we clinicians hear may make us aware of our own sexual struggles and disappointments. Many beginning therapists feel that their private sexual lives are too problematic to qualify them to help another person with this subject. Such resistance to discussing sexual matters then interacts with the patients' hesitancy to share their sexual characteristics. As a result, many well-intended therapies never get around to considering sexual issues in any significant detail.

The Five Layers of Privacy

Dealing effectively with private matters requires the clinician to appreciate the many layers that constitute the shield of sexual privacy.

---

*Mild arousal in clinical situations is sometimes referred to as "voyeuristic excitement" and is well known. Ultimately, clinicians may come to learn about their patients' internal states from their own arousal. It is not the occurrence of arousal in clinical situations that is unethical, but what the therapist may, with poor judgment, do with it.

Vocabulary Failure

When a man or a woman wants to share something private with a clinician, language often becomes a problem. Even a well-educated person may become unable to find the words to describe his or her sexual feelings or behaviors. Winks, nervous laughter, and phrases such as "You know what I mean," arise in the face of vocabulary failure. This failure has its origins in childhood when toddlers are taught the correct names for all body parts except the genitals. Boys soon learn that they have arms, hands, a nose, and a *weewee*. The genitals have emotional meanings to parents that make it difficult to call a penis a penis. Most girls grow up never hearing the word *clitoris* or the correct names for their other genital parts mentioned in their home. In many educated families, *vagina* or *vulva* are the words used to label all the genital structures. For many girls, however, the only term that is applied to their genitals is the phrase "down there." Because there is such a collusion of silence about sexual parts, feelings, and behaviors during childhood, many children come to regard their sexuality as secret when its facts, of course, are common knowledge.

By adolescence, two distinct sexual vocabularies are usually in place: an informal "dirty" set of words used for thinking and talking to peers, and an anatomically correct, frequently mispronounced, and inefficiently recalled set of words used for formal occasions. Slang terms for breast, penis, vulva, vagina, intercourse, and oral-genital stimulation number in the hundreds. The opportunity to speak about our sexual anatomy and activity, however, typically creates silence and embarrassment, not only for teenagers but for many people for all of their lives. There must be a better way of describing our sexual behavior than "messing around."

It is the task of the clinician to help the patient find a vocabulary that can be readily used without embarrassment. Usually this is the formal one that includes words like "masturbation," "mouth-genital stimulation," "penis," "ejaculation," "orgasm," and "breast." As the clinician spends more time with the patient, language tends to become slightly less formal.

Social Rules for Discussing Sexual Matters

There are three basic unwritten rules for bringing up sexual topics in polite society:

1. Don't!
2. If you must, avoid direct, plain-speaking discussion; be vague and indirect, and preferably tell a joke.
3. Do not admit to any personal sexual concerns or problems.

This suppressive cultural interpretation of proper manners keeps individuals isolated from each other in their concerns and delays the recognition of the distinction between secrecy and privacy. It also makes seeking help for a sexual concern highly anxiety-provoking because it makes one feel as though one is breaking some rule.

It is the task of the clinician to quickly rid the professional relationship of these encumbrances. The clinician and patient must be able to talk plainly, clearly, and explicitly with a minimum of innuendo and excitement. We should be able to talk about sex in a setting of privacy that finally allows for clear thinking.

Privacy Inherent in Shared Sexual Experience

This layer is formed when two consenting people share sexual behavior. What happens between them automatically becomes private without any discussion. They know the fact of their behavior is now their possession as a couple. This layer of privacy can be surrendered to the clinician who asks respectfully about it in a way that indicates that there is a valid professional reason for knowing the information.

Privacy from Sexual Partners

No matter how close we may be to a partner, there is always something about our own sexuality that is known only to us. No human being—not even the most intimate of lovers—gains a complete view of our sexual thoughts, feelings, and behaviors. What we think about during lovemaking, what images we have during masturbation, how we regarded our last sexual experience together, what we wish would occur the next time, what erotic images of our therapist we hold on to are all privacies that can instantly be made secrets by an intrusive lover or therapist. Trusted clinicians are often told about images and feelings that are kept hidden from the lover or spouse. No therapist, however, should think that she or he is to be told everything or has a right to all aspects of the patient's eroticism.

Secrets from Ourselves

Some of our sexual impulses, curiosities, and wishes run counter to our sense of sexual identity. Their appearance in our conscious minds creates anxiety. We work very hard not to know the significance of these "crazy" ideas. No matter how well we may think we know ourselves, we cannot fully grasp the source and meaning of everything we think and feel. For example, homosexual attraction and gender envy are common, well-kept secrets from heterosexual selves. Working in psychotherapy may enable a clinician to deduce such a secret from the self. This, in itself, is no reason to let the person know about it. Clinicians are expected to develop a good sense of timing because ideas that a person is not ready to hear can cause great distress and disrupt the therapeutic relationship.

Clinicians who are respectful of these five interacting layers of sexual privacy can create an environment in which sexual concerns are aired, understood, emotionally and cognitively processed, and outgrown. Usually, this clinical activity is referred to as "working through" an issue or task.

THE TASKS OF SEXUAL DEVELOPMENT

When therapists for adults, adolescents, or children are called upon to help with a sexual problem, the past of the patient is relevant. Behavior, whether problematic or not, is often subtly shaped by what has gone on before. Clinicians are not always certain, however, what preceding developmental processes are relevant to a particular current sexual problem. This section on the general tasks of sexual development is the beginning of the attempt to understand how past events and processes contribute to problematic sexual life. The key concept is the developmental task.

A *developmental task* is a necessary, unavoidable social or psychological demand for a new level of behavior. Developmental tasks do not go away. Depending on how well the task is dealt with, the person either can progress to confront newer, more sophisticated tasks that enhance self-esteem and enrich life with new opportunities or continue to struggle with the same issue, gradually eroding the person's self-confidence and opportunities. Childhood developmental tasks are relatively well-known. Here are three examples: toilet training; separation from home long enough to go to school; development of social skills. Mastery of developmental tasks is influenced both by the children themselves and their environment—that is, either the child, the parents, or the educational system can be responsible for enabling a task to be worked through or making it impossible to master. Children who fail to master these developmental landmarks become limited in their ability to learn, to participate in peer groups, and to enhance self-esteem.

There are comparable sexual developmental tasks that require both the person's and the environment's cooperation to master. The psychologically caused sexual problems of adults are often the subtle consequences of failed tasks of individual psychological and sexual development. Here are a few tasks of sexual development that range from the beginning to the end of the life cycle from which no one can hide:

1. To learn correctly about sexual anatomy and physiology and what transpires between consenting sexual partners.
2. To accept comfortably and honor our unique sexual selves.
3. To manage our sexual experiences with ourselves and with our partners without fear, victimization, or destructiveness.

4. To create the psychological and social conditions that enable us to be our most comfortable, functional sexual selves.
5. To keep sexual pleasure alive as long as the body permits.

These general tasks are different in important ways for each sex. Puberty demands different accommodations for girls than boys, for example, but the tasks of accepting the body and learning how to privately and interpersonally manage it are identical.

The extent to which people succeed at these tasks shapes their sexual experiences in life. For many people, sexual behavior is an unsatisfying ordeal, ridden with anxiety and disappointment throughout life. Others view their sexual experiences as among their very best moments of existence. Clinicians have the opportunity to hear about people in various phases of their struggles to be sexually comfortable. Many patients will have made little progress in mastering these five basic tasks. Other patients' lives illustrate the joys and richness of sexuality, so much so that the clinician feels envious. Such envy reminds the therapist that she or he has a few personal sexual developmental tasks to deal with more completely.

SUMMARY

The term *sexuality* is used in so many contexts both within and outside of the health professions that it is impossible to provide a concise definition. It is, however, an ever-present, ever-evolving, multifaceted resource of every human being that can be understood to have at least eight different contextual meanings. Each of these contexts is important for clinicians. Although privacy provides a useful protection for everyone, the confusion between privacy and secrecy prevents a wider dissemination of general sexual knowledge and the efficient satisfaction of personal curiosity. Clinicians need to recognize, respect, and skillfully work with each of the five layers of privacy in order to offer relief from sexual distress. Sexuality is shaped by biological, social, and psychological influences and evolves throughout life. The extent to which sexuality ultimately yields pleasure to the individual has much to do with how well the person masters the sexual developmental tasks.

REFERENCES

1. Kubie LS: The retreat from patients: An unanticipated penalty of the full-time system. *Archives of General Psychiatry,* 1971; 24:98–106.
2. Lear J: *Love and Its Place in Nature: A Philosophical Interpretation of Freudian Psychoanalysis.* New York, Farrar, Straus, & Giroux, 1990.
3. Person ES: *Dreams of Love and Fateful Encounters: The Power of Romantic Passion.* New York, WW Norton, 1988.

What Shapes Sexual Life?

Clinicians need to be careful about unwarranted certainty concerning sexual life. Sexual characteristics are shaped by the interactions of individual psychology, biology, interpersonal relationship, the sexual equilibrium, and culture.

Concerns about sexual life are common among all ages of the general adult population.[1,2] Assistance with these concerns is widely assumed to be available from the medical profession. But it is the mental health professional who is generally believed to be the most reliable source of knowledge about the emotional and physical aspects of sexual life.

Trainees in the mental health professions need to examine this assumption. What informs clinicians about sexuality? What bodies of knowledge, what method of information-gathering, what perspectives are supposed to be mastered in order to live up to this expectation? The answers are neither clear nor reassuring.

To be knowledgeable about sexuality, the clinician gradually accumulates a body of facts, discerns the principles of fulfilling and problematic sexual life, and eventually is able to articulate relevant unanswered questions. The clinician relies on multiple sources of learning to reach this position: personal life experiences, basic medical and social sciences, applied clinical scientific investigations, and experiences as a clinician. Each source has distinct strengths and limitations.

CAVEATS ABOUT CLINICAL WAYS OF KNOWING

Skepticism about Sexual Expertise

As could be seen from the eight definitions provided in Chapter 1, the boundaries of sexuality are not well defined. Sexuality is integral to the basic processes of life. Expertise in sexuality exists, but only in a limited way. An expert in the treatment of sexual dysfunction, for example, cannot be assumed to have a credible grasp of sexual issues outside the knowledge base of the mental health professional—for example, public policy concerning HIV transmission. This caveat can be extended to specialization within the mental health professions. For instance, some therapists who are skilled at treating psychogenic impotence know relatively little about gender disorders or paraphilia. Clinicians must critically select those who will inform them about sexual matters.

Limitations of Sexual Science and Clinical Work

Within the mental health professions, sexual knowledge stems from one of two general processes: either the measurement of data using methods that conform to general standards of science or from clinical evaluation and therapy experiences with patients with particular problems. Scientific studies of sexual topics are time-consuming, designed to be narrow in scope, difficult to fund, tedious to conduct, and, when well done, much respected. Their implications are often slowly realized by the general culture, which has only a vague appreciation that science requires replication to establish anything as fact.

Clinical approaches are faster and broader in the scope of their conclusions, are funded by patients through fees for service, and are far easier to conduct than scientific study. They are not, however, as widely respected because they are more easily influenced by the sensibilities of the therapist. Clinicians far outnumber scientists. Most of our ideas about the problems that we are called upon to deal with arise from a combination of scientific and clinical approaches; the clinical sources generally are preponderant.

Some seasoned professionals will take exception to the distinction between scientific and clinical sources. They argue that clinical work also has rigorous methods involving careful descriptions, diagnoses, hypothesis generation, and theory building and, therefore, is a form of science. Those who conceive of science as a rigorous, replicable method of learning that requires tangible measurements—even when it involves patient care—disagree. Hovering at the heart of this controversy are the philosophical questions of how we know what we know and what degree of certainty we can have about scientific and clinical conclusions.

Epistemological Conflict

These various ways of knowing, what philosophers call *epistemologies*, sometimes dramatically conflict with one another. Almost all sexual knowledge has hidden meanings to people, which can create intense, I-know-in-my-heart-I-am-correct emotions. Clinicians are not exempt. We, too, have personal values, beliefs, and notions about proper sexual feelings and behaviors. Dispassionate, objective scientific study sometimes leads to conclusions that are contrary to the clinician's beliefs. For example, a widespread quandary occurred during the early 1970s. For most of this century, the heterosexual majority within and outside of the mental health professions assumed homosexuality was an illness. There was little conflict between the mental health professionals' values that held that homosexual behaviors were abnormal and society's traditional values that people who felt and behaved this way were immoral. Some professionals, noting how homosexuals in treatment often suffered from self-loathing, kindly offered psychotherapy rather than rebuke. Then, in 1973, after considerable scientific study and debate, the American Psychiatric Association removed homosexuality from its list of mental disorders.[3] Clinicians felt a conflict between what was widely known through the culture—that homosexuals were sick—and allegiance to new scientific findings. What was previously conceived of as humane treatment began to be reconsidered as unethical professional behavior. Clinicians either had to decide which epistemology to honor, to sustain the conflict without resolution until further evidence appeared, or not to think about the contradiction.

Tensions between Personal Values and Clinical Roles

Closely related to a conflict between epistemologies is the conflict that sometimes arises between the professional's personal values and the clinical role. Usually, simply recognizing such a conflict leads to a growing comfort with the paradox and a greater understanding of the subtle issues embedded in it. Over the years, I have had only one trainee whom I regarded as impossible to help with the conflict between personal morality and clinical expectations.

> A resident physician rotating from Family Medicine to our Sexual Dysfunction Clinic was assigned to be a therapist for a cohabitating graduate student couple in their mid-twenties. His role was to evaluate and help with their concern about rapid uncontrollable ejaculation. This pattern was limiting the couple's ease and pleasure with one another. In supervision, after the first clinical hour of what seemed to be good history taking, the resident reported that he told the couple that he did not believe it is morally acceptable for unmarried people to have sexual intercourse and would not offer them treatment. Shocked, they left without further discussion. I was not only astounded at his behavior with the couple but also by the almost proud, calm manner in which he related the clinical transaction. As I tried to explain my views of unmarried people's rights to have a sexual life, his rights to conduct his life in sexual abstinence, and our clinical tradition of trying to help people understand their conflicts and dilemmas in a relatively nonjudgmental atmosphere, he firmly and politely repeated his belief that unmarried people

should not have premarital genital intimacies and then finished with, "It is not good for them!" We agreed that another specialty rotation might provide him more technical knowledge outside of sexuality. The couple was reassigned to a clinician who could separate personal values from clinical work and who did not have a righteous certainty about other people's choices.

This young clinician, of course, represents an extreme reaction, one that is not expected of those who choose to be a mental health clinician. All mental health professionals can expect, however, moments of similar conflict when they hear about the sexual tastes and behaviors of others. The most universally evocative negative reactions come about when pedophiles are seen. A far less common, but by no means rare reaction occurs when some heterosexual clinicians first hear about the homosexual behaviors of patients.

WHAT INFORMS THE CLINICIAN?

"Can you help me with this problem?" is the recurrent demand to the clinician. In order to meet this demand, clinicians must have some background knowledge. The clinician's first source of sexual knowledge arises from living as a sexual being. Many clinicians are not comfortable acknowledging this avenue of learning, for it provides no professional credentials. Actually, personal experience with sexual pleasures, concerns, and distress enables us to use our memories and associations to relate better to our patients. We need not demean our personal experience, even if it happens to be problematic, because personal sexual distress can readily become the basis of empathy and motivation for further learning.

Accumulating experience taking care of patients is a second important source of knowledge. When a clinician treats one psychogenically impotent man, for example, whatever is concluded from the therapy tends to be generalized to all similar cases. When a second man with this diagnosis is found to have differing causal circumstances, the clinician becomes more open-minded. Accumulating clinical experiences facilitates awareness of the important similarities and differences in people with the same diagnosis and allows the clinician to become curious about the next opportunity.

Sexologic science also informs the clinician. Several refereed, scholarly journals exist that present ideas that emerge from scientific study. There also is a continual stream of books that integrate scientific findings with clinical experience to generate practical approaches to sexual problems. Science is not without controversy or limitations. Scientific controversies often lead to the design of studies that are better able to answer the controversial question. Direct participation in this process can provide great pleasure for a clinician.

Outside the mental health professions, medical sciences, sociology, anthropology, general literature, history, philosophy, religion, and the media all have the potential to enrich the clinician's understanding of what influences the sexual thoughts, feelings, and behaviors of people.

CONTEXTS FOR UNDERSTANDING SEXUALITY

Explanations about the causes of sexual phenomena typically invoke forces that can be placed in one of five categories: individual psychology; biology; interpersonal relationships; the sexual equilibrium; and culture. Taken together, these categories create the usual contexts for understanding the determinants of healthy and impaired sexuality (Table 1). Taken individually, they contain enough conflicting viewpoints to occupy a scholar for a lifetime. Our current task, however, is not to consider each category in depth. Rather, it is to emphasize the idea that sexual life, to the extent it can be explained by mental health professionals, is understood using ideas taken from one or more of these five contexts.

Individual Psychology

Each person has a somewhat unique set of sexual thoughts, feelings, and behaviors. Clinicians sometimes try to explain the origins of this uniqueness from their close-in vantage point. Such attempts reflect the clinician's understanding of how minds are programmed and how they function. Clinicians who are slightly more distant from the individual patient—such as those who work primarily with couples or families—have different, more interpersonal views about how minds work. Social scientists, who have even more removed global views, are also interested in explaining how minds are programmed. Regardless of psychological ideology, individual psychology is widely agreed upon as an important place to seek an explanation for sexual life. Disagreements are bound to occur as to what is inherent in the human psyche, what is programmed by experi-

Table 1. The Usual Contexts
for Understanding Sexual Life

1. Individual psychology
2. Biology
3. Interpersonal relationships
4. Sexual equilibrium
5. Culture

ence and cultu   mental function, and how
best to explain
    For the firs   cal explanations for sexual
behaviors were   s dynamics, development,
superego-id-eg(xperiences, or internalized
images of othei   y emphasized intrapsychic
psychology to the exclusion of the world outside the person. In 1945,
Fenichel, for example, in a highly influential book,[4] discussed the origin of
sexual disorders only in terms of underlying unconscious conflict. These
conflicts were assumed to be inherent, unavoidable aspects of being
human. They were considered derivatives of the preoedipal and Oedipal
psychosexual stages of development. Today, years after psychoanalytic
theory has recognized the important role that interactions with others play
in shaping a child's conflicts, it seems strange to imagine a view of mental
life that did not include this knowledge.

Few professionals now object to the notion that there is a predictable
sequence of stages through which children and, to a lesser extent, adults
pass which are enriched or disturbed by the quality of their significant
relationships, experiences of living in a family, and years of participation in
a particular subculture. The thinking about etiology is far broader today
that it was in the past. During the last 30 years, each major theory—
psychoanalytic, behavioral, systems—has fertilized the others. The current
explanations for sexual symptoms are no longer rigidly linked to any particular theory.

I think of the four contexts that follow as additional mechanisms for
the sexual programming of the mind. They are the shaping influences on
the sexual psyche that arise from outside the person's inherent psychology.

Biology

From the vast subject of biology, I want to emphasize four forces that
subtly contribute to individual psychology: sexual temperament, aging,
organic disease, and psychological control of physiology. First, there is the
matter of sexual endowment. Babies begin to display certain characteristics
early in life that are consistently present for years when they have been
prospectively tracked throughout childhood and adolescence.[5] These traits
are referred to as *temperament*. Although the original pioneering work on
temperament did not included sexual traits, it is an easy conceptual step to
formulate a sexual temperament. For example, what we understand as
femininity has been noted in many gender-disturbed boys less than 18
months of age. For many of these boys, biology may be the best explanation for the intensity and persistence of the femininine traits.[6] The same
may be true for early intense masculinity traits in girls. How pre- and

ent creates temperamental predispositions to
ι to accepted notions of appropriate male and
ious.

al, aspect of sexual temperament is the matter
ty of the internal push to behave sexually. With
ted most clearly during adolescence, the pos-
iological processes contribute to events that are
played out years later. Epidemiologists have noted that most teenagers can
be divided into three groups by the frequency of masturbation: a small
percentage of those who have little-to-no masturbation or other sexual
outlets, a similar percentage of those with at least daily rates, and the vast
majority with once-to-several orgasms per week.[7] The significance of sex
drive as a temperamental endowment may be great for males because it has
been shown that a higher sex drive earlier in life predicts a longer, more
sexually functional sexual life in the latter stages of the life cycle, whereas a
low sex drive early in life predicts a shorter span of sexual behavior and a
higher prevalence of dysfunction.[8] Quantitative studies of drive in females
do not exist, but women are certainly not immune to the biological influences on sex drive. Most women are able to specify a time during their
menstrual cycle when their sexual drive manifestations tend to occur. Science has yet to be able to discern the neuroendocrine explanations for this
common phenomenon.

The second biological shaping force is the process of aging. The sexual
response system, an integrated neuroendocrine-vascular physiological organization, has maximal efficiency in youth and slowly deteriorates decade
by decade. By their seventh decade, many women and men can be very
clear about the changes in their sexual capacities that have gradually become apparent during the previous 20 years.[9] The deterioration of biological sexual capacities means that psychological adversity can be more sexually disruptive among elderly women and men.

The third and usually most obvious biological shaping force consists of
the organic diseases and medications that impair sexual drive, arousal
capacities, and orgasmic attainment. These illnesses and their treatments
are most common during the latter half of the life cycle, when, simultaneously, the gradual, subtle effects of sexual aging are lessening the
intensity and frequency of drive, the ease and reliability of arousal, and the
facility to attain orgasm.

A fourth relevant biological explanation for sexual problems involves
the actual physiological mechanisms whereby desire, arousal, and orgasm
are muted or paralyzed by psychological dilemma or conflict. Although
many sexual problems are considered psychogenic, the mind in conflict
operates through unknown brain mechanisms. Science may be heading in
the direction of ascertaining this psychogenic mechanism in terms of neurotransmission.

Interpersonal Relationship

Partner sexual behavior is conducted within a broader nonsexual context that subtly shapes what is felt, said, and done sexually. Few sexually active people have to live very long before they discover the power that nonsexual issues have in fashioning their sexual experiences. In a comfortable relationship, the most important factor that limits sexual behavior is anger over unresolved nonsexual matters. Other feelings, such as guilt, anxiety, or fear of communicating, that derive from participation in a relationship also can limit what is felt and done sexually.

Once in a committed relationship, many adults intuitively understand that their behavior always has implications and meanings for their partner. Many people lie or keep secrets because they accurately grasp what these meanings will be to their partner. Decisions to behave in certain ways—for example, to refuse to be civil to a spouse's family, to continue drinking, or to half-heartedly care for the children—can create interpersonal havoc that makes sexual pleasure impossible.

Relationships are living entities which can be sustained, enhanced, or crippled. Sexual problems sometimes can only be understood by grasping the nature of the partners' nonsexual interactions. Therapy for such sexual problems requires the clinician to be skillful with nonsexual matters.

The living entity of a marriage can be crippled by the decision of a spouse to have an extramarital affair. Whether or not the partner becomes directly aware of the infidelity, the emotional tenor of the marital relationship may change and create sexual problems that cannot be understood except with the knowledge of the partner's secret.

Sexual Equilibrium

The least recognized influence on sexual responsiveness is the sexual equilibrium. The sexual equilibrium is a balance of the interaction of the sexual capacities of each partner and how each partner regards those capacities. This balance either creates sexual comfort or discomfort. It operates as follows. Each partner brings a number of traits to the bedroom—for example, a weak or strong interest in behaving sexually; ease or difficulty becoming aroused; ease or difficulty attaining orgasm (Table 2). Each person perceives and reacts to these sexual traits. That reaction is seen or felt by the partner. One partner may be induced to relax or to be made anxious by what the other partner's reaction is perceived to be. One partner might simultaneously react to multiple traits of the other. The sum of these interactions is referred to as the *sexual equilibrium*.

The sexual equilibrium is a useful concept in explaining why a person with a consistent set of sexual characteristics—for instance, rapid ejaculation or slowness to be aroused—can become dysfunctional with one part-

*Table 2. Two Types of Interactions Constituting
the Sexual Equilibrium*

Partner A	Partner B
Sexual identity components ⟷	Sexual identity components
Gender	Gender
Orientation	Orientation
Intention	Intention
Sexual function components ⟷	Sexual function components
Desire	Desire
Arousal	Arousal
Orgasm	Orgasm
Sexual satisfaction ⟷	Sexual satisfaction

ner and have a happy functional sexual life with another. The sexual equilibrium refers only to the balance of perceptions and attitudes about the sexual traits and the actual interaction of the two people. It is highly influenced by the hidden meanings that these sexual traits have for each person. For some women, rapid ejaculation of the partners means, "Dammit, I will not have a chance to enjoy intercourse." For others, it means, "He finds me very exciting." For some men, a woman's pattern of orgasm that is stimulated only by clitoral stimulation means, "I am an inadequate lover" or "She does not really love me." For other men, the same pattern means, "I love it when she attains orgasm." The difference between these initial attitudes may determine whether the couple continues to have a sexual life at all, and sometimes whether they continue as a couple. Some clinicians prefer to consider the sexual equilibrium as a subcategory of the interpersonal context—the subcategory that confines itself to sexual traits. The sexual equilibrium is discussed in greater detail in Chapter 7.

Culture

That culture shapes us is irrefutable. However, the process by which cultural values, attitudes, and beliefs become incorporated into our psyches is not well understood. The social sciences are devoted to illustrating that what a person feels, thinks, and does is influenced by cultural forces stemming from participation in family, subcultural, regional, and national life.

When it comes to sexual life, culture defines the roles that men and women play. Vocations, emotional expressiveness, styles of femininity and masculinity, education about sexual matters, the degree of giving and receiving of sexual pleasures, responsibility for contraception, standards for the expected duration of intercourse, frequency of intercourse, whether homosexuality is a sin, premarital virginity, and women's right to expect sexual pleasure are all partial reflections of cultural influences.[10] Sociologists and anthropologists provide a shocking perspective for those who assume that most of psychology is inherent in the psyche. What we take for granted in our culture as natural actually differs dramatically from society to society. Two examples follow:

Anthropologist Gilbert Herdt has delineated an instructive style of acculturating boys into heterosexuality among the Sambia of New Guinea.[11] After a prolonged period of living only with women, boys are placed in the company of adolescent and adult males. Among the methods for learning how to be a man in this isolated tribe is the expectation for daily fellation of their elders. The culture interprets this behavior as necessary for the development of manhood which includes heterosexual behavior. Cross-dressing and homosexual behaviors do not occur among the men.

Sociologists Reiss and Reiss[10] have tried to illustrate the power of patriarchal social arrangements to shape our sexual experiences by describing a hypothetical society called *Matriarchia*. In Matriarchia, women dominate every major institution; there it is natural that boys and men grow up realizing that they have less power. Here are their words:

> In such a society what would men do to protect the little power they have? They would feel that their sexual attractiveness was one of the few assets they had that was valued by the more powerful group of women, and they would play those cards very carefully. Women could easily use a man sexually and quickly turn from one man to another. So a man would have to be careful not to squander his one source of influence. Men would try to make women assure them in some way that they are not being used. Men would be far less sexually assertive. They would see sex as a service to women. Women would not just sit by and let men use their masculine wiles to lure them into sexual bargaining. If they felt that men were not treating them right, some of them would gang up on a man and force him to perform whatever sexual acts they desired. Women would demand faithful partners but also insist that some men be available to them for quick pleasure. To insure male sexual restraint, women would connect sexuality to romantic love for men and tell men that when they are swept away by love for a particular woman, then and only then, can they enjoy themselves sexually. Any man that violated that romantic code would be labelled a "slut." But, of course, ruling women would not place any such negative labels on themselves. (pp. 97–98)

THOMAS—A CASE HISTORY

Much of what we clinicians come to think of as the dynamics or etiology of a situation is just deduction and speculation based on combinations of ideas taken from these five contexts. No single clinician can be expected to grasp the exact extent that these contexts have shaped a person's sexual problems. This inability is not to be demeaned. As the clinician spends time trying to understand a patient, the problem is often resolved. I diagnosed Thomas as having psychogenic erectile dysfunction and retarded ejaculation. Can you perceive how forces from each of the five contexts might be said to have shaped his problem?

Thomas is a 56-year-old financially secure widower, a high-level executive, father of one married daughter, an excellent dancer and golfer. Six months previously, after 3 years of almost steady deterioration with breast cancer, his 51-year-old socially prominent wife died. Left alone with a big house, he kept himself busy at work, with work-related travel, and social engagements with his many acquaintances. His grief was largely anticipatory and after two frenetic, but miserable, months, he was no longer sad, preoccupied with his wife's memory, or unable to fully concentrate. "It is over! I just don't like to be sad. I've had enough of it!" When his daughter wanted to talk about memories of her mother, he abruptly cut her off with "We'll have none of that!"

Thomas, always conservatively dressed during his 15 therapy sessions, is a well-organized, neat, meticulously clean, rational man, who insists upon immaculateness in his office and home. In his early meetings with me, he spoke disdainfully of himself as a "good boy." Not permitted to swear by his mother and his wife, he now enjoys peppering his speech with four-letter words. Previously unflinchingly polite, he now occasionally demonstrates irritation. Each time, for example, when I asked about his family background, he bristled and overruled me, "Not relevant!"

He grudgingly allowed me a glimpse of his marriage after telling me that the problem is only in the present. They had no sexual contact since her cancer diagnosis. For the decade prior to her illness, their frequency of quick, mutually orgasmic missionary-style intercourse had dwindled to approximately every three weeks. "I don't really know why except that our life together was not particularly emotionally exciting."

Thomas passionately spoke of being tired of his former life. He no longer wanted to attend benefits for charity, to circulate among the right people, or to behave properly. He viewed his widowhood as his first opportunity to do the things that were unavailable to him as a faithful married man for 30 years.

Thomas was a highly eligible bachelor. Nice looking, trim, not concerned about money, in excellent physical health, unencumbered by children, socially at ease, he had no trouble filling his life with interested women. Although his early dates were with women from his former social circles, he was quickly "smitten" by an 11-year-younger, high school educated, ungrammatical, voluptuous, sexually provocative divorcée with three children who "didn't have two nickels to rub together." At every sexual opportunity with her, however, despite her intense efforts to help, Thomas was unable to obtain an erection. "What is wrong with me? This woman is perfect—she has a lovely face, wonderful breasts, a small waist, she is very clean, yet here is Thomas with nothing between his legs!" She suggested he see a doctor.

Thomas did not feel comfortable masturbating at his age. When he occasionally did, he was puzzled by his consistent ability to obtain a full erection and a strong orgasm while thinking about this woman's perfect body. His morning erections were also full several times per week.

Thomas agreed with my summary that he seemed to be at war with himself. His affair with this woman, whom he only saw alone, was a social embarrassment to him. His emotional attraction to her seemed to gather its power from his wish to escape the restraint of his upper-class proper life-style. "She is so down to earth, so basic, she swears like a trooper," he chortled. "I think I love her! I want to help her, see her, talk to her, touch her. Am I crazy? This is a disaster. You gotta help me!"

For several months, Thomas's social life continued with several charming, attractive, educated women for whom he lacked all erotic desire. During these months, he saw or talked to his "love" several times a week. His dating stopped while he became involved in a 3-week intense relationship with a middle-class woman who frightened him by her quick devotion to him, despite his erection problems ("Don't use the word *impotent*, doctor, I hate it!"). Another intense, but longer relationship ensued with a woman who first warned him of her sexual troubles stemming from her sexual abuse with her father. "I have my own form of sexual problems—widower's impotence," he told her. His erections began to recover within this relationship as they spent whole weekends together in his house, away from his friends. Her ingenuity and determination delighted Thomas and helped him to relax. Their exchange of oral-genital stimulation provided him pleasures he never experienced in marriage. He was unable to ejaculate in her presence, however, despite her devoted efforts.

This partner deduced that Thomas's primary interest in her was as a sex partner about the same time she suspected that Thomas was emotionally involved with another woman. She was greatly disappointed, but calm. Thomas then pulled away from her because "Her depression is a burden and I don't need any more troubles."

On one of his out-of-town business trips, he met a long divorced, childless businesswoman in her early forties with whom, unlike the other people he had been out with, he could talk at length about himself. He loved being with her and was not ashamed to be seen anywhere with her. He experienced her as beautiful, warm, emotionally stable, and intelligent. There was no need to hide her. Despite the fact that he felt he was slowly falling in love with her, he still tried unsuccessfully to have sex with his first "love." As his out-of-town relationship progressed, however, he only saw this first woman platonically.

Thomas and his new love had a long wonderful vacation together marked by two episodes of unpleasantness that created panicky feelings for him. He was worried either because he might lose her or that she was not as stable as he thought and he ought to end the relationship. On two occasions, he reported that her mood suddenly turned from wonderful to foul for no reason. When she could tell him what she was angry about, he became confused. Twice, while sitting in hotel lobbies, his eyes fixed on another woman and he lost track of their conversation as though he was mesmerized. He could not believe that his glance was anything like she described—that is, an endless stare that simultaneously insulted his partner and the other woman. In defense, he reminded her that on the first occasion, they began agreeing at how unusual and lovely looking the woman was. Otherwise, their trip was wonderful. He felt he was making progress in getting closer to ejaculation but was not there yet. When they had another long opportunity to be together, she continued to be concerned about his lack of ejaculation, but primarily because she was having a great sexual experience with him, she wanted him to feel the intensity for himself. Unlike the previous two partners, his ejaculation did not become the object of their sexual interaction. He thought that even without orgasm, his sexual experiences with her were wonderful. He reaffirmed he loved her, wanted her to give up her job and move in with him, and soon to marry him. As she was seriously considering giving up her life in another city, and he became convinced that she genuinely loved him, he began to ejaculate regularly. His understanding of his return to full sexual function and pleasure was stated to me as though I knew this all along: "I know it is because I love her, of course. I couldn't ejaculate with the others because there was no love there."

She moved in with him and was pleasantly working to establish a social and vocational life for herself when she became deeply distressed over Thomas's staring again. When I saw panicky Thomas, his focus was on his innocence and what possibly could be wrong with this wonderful woman. When I saw her alone, however, nothing seemed wrong with her. She was wondering about the meaning of his staring at other women's breasts and skirts and what it portended about a life together. She was trying to answer several questions. "Does he not love me?" "Will he soon be unfaithful?" "Should I go back home?" A few days later when I saw the couple together, she had spoken to his daughter about her worry and found out that this trait had embarrassed her and her mother several times.

Thomas was contrite, apologetic, and agitated that he might lose her over what he considered his ordinary male activities. When he was confronted with the fact that his wife had also criticized him for this same rudeness, he blushed and nodded that he remembered. I spoke of his repressed sexual self, alluded to the sexual freedom that followed his wife's death, and the need to allow himself to know about his bodily interest in women so he could control its expression. His fiancée felt reassured that Thomas was basically the good person she initially met and agreed to marry.

One year later, Thomas, now living together with his fiancée in another city, called for a referral to a marital therapist. "Sex is fine, couldn't be better, no problem with it whatsoever, but the problem of looking has recurred." They are not yet married, in part because they wanted to give his married adult daughter more time to adjust to their relationship.

SUMMARY

Complexity prevents us from knowing exactly what shapes our particular sexual characteristics. Five forces interact to determine our experience as a sexual person: individual psychology, biology, interpersonal relationship, the sexual equilibrium, and culture. This complexity can be dangerous for clinicians and scientists who long for well-established facts and irrefutable principles. Differing ways of knowing—clinical experience versus scientific study—often result in conflicting conclusions about sexual issues. And because sexual behaviors are inextricably linked to personal and cultural values, professionals often find it difficult to agree upon what is normal, what the ultimate source of a problem is, and which sexual expert to trust. Clinicians are on safer ground when they appreciate the sources of their knowledge and the limits of their understanding. Despite the problems about knowing about sexual life, the pursuit of understanding sexuality can be intellectually enriching and clinically useful. The evolution of one person's sexual problem is recounted in order to illustrate how the five interacting forces shape the dynamics of sexual experience.

REFERENCES

1. Frank E, Anderson B, Rubinstein D: Frequency of sexual dysfunction in "normal" couples. *New England Journal of Medicine,* 1978; 299:111–115.
2. Schein M, Zyzanski S, Levine SB, Dickman R, Alegomagno S: The frequency of sexual problems among family practice patients. *Family Practice Research Journal,* 1988; 7(3):122–134.
3. Bayer RV: *Homosexuality and American Psychiatry: The Politics of Diagnosis.* New York, Basic Books, 1981.
4. Fenichel O: *Psychoanalytic Theory of Neuroses.* New York, WW Norton, 1945.
5. Chess A, Thomas S: Genesis and evolution of behavioral disorders from infancy to early adult life. *American Journal of Psychiatry,* 1984; 141(1):1–9.
6. Green R: *"The Sissy Boy Syndrome" and the Development of Male Homosexuality.* New Haven, Yale University Press, 1987.
7. Kinsey AC, Pomeroy WB, Martin CE: *Sexual Behavior in the Human Male.* Philadelphia, WB Sanders, 1948.
8. Martin CE: Factors affecting sexual functioning in 60–79 married males. *Archives of Sexual Behavior,* 1981; 10:399–420.
9. Bachmann GA, Lieblum SR: Sexuality in sexagenarian women. *Maturitas,* 1991; 13:43–50.
10. Reiss IL, Reiss HM: *An End to Shame: Shaping Our Next Sexual Revolution.* Buffalo, Prometheus Books, 1990.
11. Herdt G: *Guardian of the Flutes: Idioms of Masculinity.* New York, McGraw-Hill, 1981.

The Psychological Organization of Our Sexual Selves

The mind functions as though it is constantly integrating seven sexual components. These components guide our understanding of sexual health and distress.

Neuroscientists have recently become interested in the relationship between the structure and physiology of the brain and sexual psychology. As progress is made, some aspects of the ideas discussed here may be eventually more fundamentally understood. For now, however, knowledge of sexual anatomy does not extend much beyond the recognition that there are internal and external genital structures, secondary sex characteristics, hypothalamic nuclei, and neuropathways that mediate their function. When it comes to basic explanations of sexual physiology, there is a comparable dearth of in-depth reliable knowledge.

Sexual psychology is another matter. Each person seems to have a discernible mental sexual organization. This "anatomy" is manifested by thoughts and feelings that order our perceptions and motivate our sexual responses and behaviors. It defines who we are, who our partners will be, what we want to do with them, and the degree of desire for, comfort with, and pleasure in sexual activities. Although science may not be able to describe how the brain creates sexuality, our "anatomy" has two major divisions: sexual identity and sexual function.

SEXUAL IDENTITY

Sexual identity is a composite of three important dimensions of personal experience: *gender, orientation,* and *intention.* Because most people have superficially similar conventional sexual identities, they consider themselves "normal" and do not give much thought to the subject. Their experience contrasts with those who are uncertain about their sexual identities. Individuals who are uncertain may spend much energy in their early lives worrying about their gender, orientation, or intention.

Conventional and unconventional are not synonyms for normal and abnormal. *Conventional* refers to sensing the self to be more or less like the usual portrayals of others, whereas *unconventional* denotes the opposite. The distinction between normality and abnormality is a political, value-laden subject about which there are many opinions within and outside the mental health professions. Like it or not, clinicians must return to the subject because we are entrusted with making diagnoses and recommending and conducting therapies for abnormalities. A detailed understanding of sexual identity is needed to perform these activities.

In this section, our purpose is to appreciate the variety of sexual identities that exist among human beings and to understand that this diversity is contributed to by differences in its three dimensions.

Sexual Identity as an Evolving Mosaic

Sexual identity usually appears to have two characteristics—*homogeneity* and *constancy.* Neither is absolutely correct, however. Its illusory aspects can be understood through an analogy to art. When we stand at a usual distance from a recognizable painting, it has a cohesiveness that enables our brains to appreciate the image. When we move closer to it, the image loses its wholeness and we are more apt to be able to appreciate its components—brushstrokes, dots, lines, pieces of glass, and so forth. Similarly, when we look at the ordinary woman, she usually appears feminine to us, acts as though she is heterosexual, and does nothing to contradict our assumption that she wants to make love by having intercourse. When we move closer, as clinicians can, our scrutiny may reveal some unexpected elements: masculinity, homoerotic interest, or fascinations with sadomasochism, for example. These subtleties of gender, orientation, and intention often coexist with other conventional dimensions of sexual identity in the woman's privacy.

Sexual identity is formed in childhood and evolves during adolescence and young adulthood. What is created by the first half of life usually persists. There are some individuals who experience a major evolution in their sexual identity in their middle or later years, however. One of my patients, after living a seemingly comfortable life as a gender conventional, bisexual man, decided to live as a woman when he was 42 years old.

The Erotic and Sexual Realms

Sexual identity has two aspects—a *subjective*, psychological, unseen realm and an *objective*, behavioral, visible realm. In this book, the suffix

"-erotic" will be used to refer only to mental phenomena that belong to the subjective, private psychological realm, whereas the suffix "-sexual" will be used to refer only to behaviors involving the self or partners (Table 3). Clinical work allows access to the subjective, erotic realm. Scientific work tends to be preoccupied with the more quantifiable behavioral sexual realm.

Gender

Gender is the experience of oneself or another person as male or female, and masculine and feminine. It is different from "sex," which refers to the biological distinction between females and males. *Sex* refers to such bodily matters as vagina, penis, lactation, and ejaculation. *Gender* refers to the psychological experience of these anatomical and physiological distinctions. Gender is the first aspect of sexual identity to form and is usually demonstrable by age 2. It is probably created by biologic, social, and psychological forces (see Chapter 7), but for clinical purposes, gender identity in childhood functions as though it is the result of answers to the following five questions:

1. Am I a girl or a boy?
2. Can I accept this label?
3. Do I like this body with its distinctive genital parts?
4. Can I find comfort in my family's prescriptions for conventional girl and boy behaviors?
5. Can I accept the idea I will grow up to be a woman or a man?

Gender role behavior differs according to how these questions are answered. Early in life, gender role behaviors provide a window to the gender identifications the child is making. A 3-year-old boy who thinks of himself as a girl, rejects the idea that he is destined to grow up to be a man, pretends he does not have a penis, and does not want to play with boy toys usually first demonstrates his gender identity through behaviors within the family. Family members find meaning in these behaviors and react to them with varying degrees of comfort or alarm. Much later in life, when the child has learned how to mask what he feels in order to please his family, his

Table 3. The "Anatomy" of Sexual Identity

Dimension	Psychological aspect	Behavioral aspect
Gender	Gender identity	Gender role
Orientation	Erotic object choice	Sexual object choice
Intention	Preferred erotic imagery	Preferred sexual act

subjective, erotic images of himself may be feminine even though his gender role behaviors are sufficiently masculine and do not disturb his family.

The vast majority of children breeze through the developmental task of accepting their biologic sex and adapting to the cultural expectations of conventional feminine or masculine behaviors. Even among these children, however, unconventional answers sometimes are considered. Children playing house do not always want to play mother or father just because they are a girl or a boy. "What is it like to be the other sex?" is not just a question for playwrights and philosophers. It is a reasonable question about which many girls and boys are curious. After the young child has satisfied this curiosity and is able to answer these five questions in a conventional manner, she or he is likely to have no memory of ever being interested in the question. Professionals sometimes refer the result of the completion of this developmental task as the establishment of a *core gender identity*. Core gender identity can be feminine, for example, regardless of the biological sex of the child.

Conventional people have a core gender identity that follows from their biologic sex. Their subjective—that is, erotic—and objective—that is, sexual—realms of gender are usually consonant with one another. This is particularly so for most social purposes. But, in terms of deeply private, conscious experience, conventional women and men often sense themselves to be like the opposite sex in some ways.*

Later in life, gender identity can be more clearly recognized as: (1) comfort with the body as belonging to its biological sex; and (2) interest in and comfort with whatever the culture labels as appropriate feminine and masculine behaviors. Private feelings of unmasculinity or unfemininity are a common part of the subjective lives of many people. Although modern societies are redefining acceptable masculine and feminine styles of dress, recreation, relationships, emotional expression patterns, vocation, and political rights, it is important for clinicians to refuse to assume that conventional gender role behaviors predict that a person's gender identity is likewise conventional.

Orientation

The second dimension of sexual identity also can be best understood by separating its subjective and behavioral realms. It is likely that orientation begins to emerge prior to puberty and undergoes further elaboration with puberty and adolescent and young adult experience. Erotic orientation derives from private information and, therefore, the clinician must inquire: What is your orientation? What leads you to say that? Which sex

*Carl Jung, in a different context, considered each person to have feminine and masculine parts of the self, which he called the *anima* and the *animus*.

attracts you? Is this attraction exclusive? Which sex do you daydream about and use in masturbation scenarios? What has the sex been of those you have had crushes on or fallen in love with? These questions elicit an understanding of the person's differential arousal responses to each sex. The answers enable the clinician to think of a person's erotic orientation as heteroerotic, homoerotic, bierotic, or anerotic.

In keeping with a longstanding psychiatric tradition, the term *object* is used when one wants to refer to a generic human being in a theoretical sense. Orientation is based on the sex of the object choice. A male who is attracted to males is said, for instance, to have males as an object choice.*

Unlike its erotic realm, behavioral orientation is not defined by thoughts, attractions, romantic feelings, and arousing images. Rather, it is defined by the gender of a person's partners and the ability to be aroused with them. Although some people are exclusively heterosexual or homosexual, and a few are bisexual, others are only predominantly heterosexual or homosexual.

Kinsey and his colleagues devised two scales that ranked people between zero (exclusively heterosexual) and 6 (exclusively homosexual).[1] They applied one scale to fantasy and the other to behavior. I have taken the liberty to use the language distinctions of -erotic and -sexual to designate how this scale might be conceptually used (Table 4). For practical purposes, Kinsey categories of 2 and 4 are difficult to identify.

Usually, a person's orientation is fixed for life by early adulthood. An important exception to this is found in a small minority of women who, although they previously considered themselves to be heteroerotic, discover their homoeroticism in their late twenties or older, and then behave homosexually with pleasure and comfort for the first time. It is not unusual for individuals to go to college considering themselves to be conventional only to have a number of erotic and sexual experiences that lead them to reconsider their orientation.

Intention

The third dimension of sexual identity delineates what a person wants to do during sexual behavior. Conventional intentions are dominated by peaceful motivations to give and receive pleasure without pain, victimization, dehumanization, or humiliation. This is sometimes summarized as *peaceable mutuality.* Conventional intentions leave much room for a variety of transient erotic images, experimentation, and discovery of the many ways to behave sexually. Clinicians often have their attention drawn to sexual images or behaviors that are consistently dominated by sadism,

---

*"Object" is a most unpleasant, dehumanizing term that appears in many professional writings and discussions.

Table 4. The Modified Kinsey Scales

Rank	Behavioral description	Fantasy description
0	Exclusively heterosexual	Exclusively heteroerotic
1	Predominantly heterosexual	Predominantly heteroerotic
2	Heterosexual but more than incidental homosexual behavior	Heteroerotic but more incidental homoerotic arousal
3	Bisexual	Bierotic
4	Homosexual but more than incidental heterosexual behavior	Homoerotic but more than incidental heteroerotic arousal
5	Predominantly homosexual	Predominantly homoerotic
6	Exclusively homosexual	Exclusively homoerotic

masochism, exhibitionism, voyeurism, or genital sex with children. Clinicians less frequently encounter people with images and behaviors that involve interactions with inanimate materials—such as leather, silk, or shoes—that seem more important than the person who is wearing them.

In the intention dimension of sexual identity, the relationship between the erotic and the sexual is more variable than in the gender and orientation dimensions. Most unconventional images do not get directly acted out in behavior.

A Vocabulary Exercise

The following descriptions of unconventional sexual identities can now be understood in terms of the erotic and sexual aspects of the three dimensions of sexual identity. Each dimension of identity described in these examples should be traced to a location in Table 3.

1. He is a homoerotic asexual.
2. She is a homoerotic bisexual.
3. He has a strong feminine gender identity but his gender role behaviors are conventionally masculine.
4. She is a heteroerotic asexual.
5. The patient is preoccupied with masochistic and sadistic imagery but his only partner sexual behavior is through obscene phone calls or calls to the sex hotline.
6. She is a masculine-feeling, masculine-looking woman who is planning to begin living as a man soon. Her erotic orientation exclusively involves women in fantasy. She has only been sexually

active with women partners. Her erotic intentions are sadistic but she practices peaceable mutuality.

7. He is slightly effeminate in manner and wears clothes that seem more unisexual than masculine or feminine. He recalls being called a "sissy" for many years, preferred to play with girls, and hated any rough-and-tumble activities. He says he has had no sexual experiences but he sometimes masturbates to images of being tied up and tortured by strong men who force him to perform oral sex on them.

SEXUAL FUNCTION

In adolescence and beyond, as we discover our capacities for sexual function, partner sexual experiences help us to refine our sense of competence as sexual persons. This is often spoken of as either enhancing or diminishing femininity or masculinity—that is, *gender identity*. Sexual function has important contributions to make to female and male gender identity, but sexual function should not be confused with sexual identity.

Sexual function also has three major dimensions: *desire, arousal,* and *orgasm.* Together, they comprise our sexual response system. Each dimension is fundamentally psychosomatic—that is, each is shaped by biological, social, and psychological factors. Table 5 delineates the sexual function components into their subjective and objective aspects.

Sexual Desire

The correct diagnosis of many complicated sexual problems rests upon the understanding that sexual desire is the amalgamation of three concep-

Table 5. The Sexual Function Components

Dimension	Subjective aspect	Objective aspect
Desire	Genital sensations; erotic imagery; willingness to have sex; wishes and expectations	Initiation of sexual behavior
Arousal	Localized sensual skin and genital pleasures	Vaginal lubrication or penile erection
Orgasm	Intense brief explosion of genital pleasure	Pelvic contractions or ejaculation

tually separate components. Indeed, clinical progress in the treatment of sexual dysfunctions can be charted by the appreciation of the important differences in the components of desire.[2]

1. *Sexual drive.* A brain-based generator or sexual feelings exists that is known to have an important anatomic localization as a nucleus in the anterior medial preoptic area of the hypothalamus.[3] This center, too small to be localized with current clinical radiological techniques, is known as the *sexual drive center* in lower animals. It has numerous connections to the limbic system and cortex. When it is surgically destroyed, animals do not behave sexually. When it is biochemically stimulated, animals behave sexually more frequently. Understanding of the neuroendocrine factors that allow sexual drive to manifest itself in humans is still empirical, but it is clear that testosterone is necessary for sexual drive intensity in both sexes. A host of drugs are known to dampen sexual drive and to interfere with human sexual expression. Sexual drive is manifested by one or more of the following clinically observable subjective and objective phenomena:

(a) genital tingling from small degrees of clitoral and penile tumescence;
(b) erotic preoccupations, fantasies, or mental rehearsals for sexual behaviors;
(c) increased erotic responsiveness to others in the environment; and
(d) planning for and seeking sexual behaviors involving self-stimulation through masturbation or partner-related sexual activity.

Sexual drive results in early sexual arousal. Some clinicians refer to it as a central excitement which makes an individual more responsive to external erotic clues and sexual interactions. I have thought of sexual drive as spontaneous endogenous arousal.

2. *Sexual motivation.* In order to have sexual relations with a partner, individuals have to be willing to bring their bodies to the partner for the physical interaction. This willingness is taken for granted by most people with sexual drive. For them, either drive and motivation seem to be the same phenomenon or drive invariably motivates them to behave sexually. Clinicians see people in two other situations that emphasize the separateness of drive and motivation to behave with a partner:

(a) patients who have little drive but bring their bodies regularly to sexual interactions;
(b) patients with robust drive manifestations who will not bring their bodies to their partner.

Sexual motivation ranges between two polarities: strong motives to make love with a particular partner and strong motives to avoid lovemaking with a particular partner. In couples without sexual problems, each partner's motives to make love may change quickly in response to many current factors. In dysfunctional sexual lives, motives to avoid lovemaking often have a grip on people. The complexities, nuances, and clinical challenges of sexual motivation far exceed those of sexual drive.

3. *Sexual wish.* Powerful expectations about sexual behavior exist in people apart from their experience of sexual drive and motive. These expectations reflect ideas that derive from affiliations with various social groups—such as age group, race, economic class, ethnic group, religious affiliation, and vocation. These many affiliations and identifications provide us with ideas that shape the expression of desire. Sexual wishes or expectations can be for or against sexual behavior.

Strong expectations can translate into a sense of entitlement to have sexual intercourse at a certain frequency. "I'm a 33-year-old normal woman and I expect to be able to have intercourse with my husband at least twice a week!" "I'm only 15 years old and I do not expect to have intercourse yet, I would like to, but I don't think I should." Age, parental relationships, church affiliation, and ethnic ideas of the importance of virginity may create in both sexes a strong expectation not to have intercourse. Middle-aged and older adults sometimes find their personal expectations to avoid intercourse as being ludicrously Victorian, but they, nonetheless, may initially delay a much desired experience until they think about and work through their wishes not to have intercourse outside of marriage.

The effect of conscience can be seen in the wish component of sexual desire. But sexual wishes, expectations, or cognitions contain forces other than conscience: they reflect the person's identifications with social groups. "I am a red-blooded 65-year-old American man and I want to have intercourse. Please, fix me, doctor, so that I can once again enjoy this." An 88-year-old man taught me about the need to separate wish from drive and motive. When I asked him if he had sexual desire, he replied as did the red-blooded American—with pride and entitlement. He, however, had not had any sexual contact with his wife for 3 years. When I asked about his experience with sexual drive, he laughed and said he hadn't felt that way in 20 years. He heard that there was a way to restore men sexually and he wanted it.

Sexual desire is the end product of the interaction of these three complexities: a biological force called *drive*, a psychological force called *motive*, and a social force called *wish*. When these forces all point in the same positive direction, arousal can be easy. But, they often conflict with one another to create a weakened desire whose comings and goings may be baffling.

Sexual Arousal

Arousal is an emotion that is triggered by erotic stimuli. Like other emotions, it has an invariable programmed genetic sequence of physiological events that consist of messages from the brain to the vascular system.

As this emotion is sustained or intensified in women, blood is rerouted from storage sites in the mesentery to the pelvic organs. The walls of the vagina become redder, warmer, and moister, the clitoris enlarges, the labia minora become darker and thicker, and the uterus elevates slightly. In males, the penis elongates and becomes firm, the testes enlarge and move up to the perineum, and the scrotum becomes smaller. Intense arousal is more than a genital vascular phenomenon, but the other changes are not as invariable. There are both early relaxing and later tensing muscular responses, respiratory rate changes, and transient increases in blood pressure and heart rate as this emotion nears triggering off the next major physiologic event—orgasm.

Psychologically, sexual arousal requirements are relatively unique from person to person. Not only does the person's sexual identity dictate different conditions for arousal, but additional requirements of suitable conditions under which to make love come into being. Once these conditions are met and two people behave sexually, the physiological changes are predictable.

Sexual Orgasm

Orgasm attracts most of the attention, but it is only the dramatic step in the psychophysiologic sexual response sequence. It is a reflexive series of preprogrammed events triggered by reaching a neurophysiologic threshold of arousal. In women, these events last up to 20 seconds.[4] They begin with a subjective sensation followed by rhythmic contractions of the muscles of the outer third of the vagina. Vaginal contractions may also be synchronous with contractions of the myometrium and the anus.

In men, orgasm may be slightly shorter. It begins with a subjective state of pleasure called the *state of ejaculatory inevitability.* This corresponds to the contractions of smooth muscles in the prostate, seminal vesicles, and vas deferens which fill the prostatic urethra with semen and spermatozoa. The urethra is stretched by this fluid, the external bladder sphincter relaxes, and the bulbocavernosus and ischiocavernosus muscles contract to propel the ejaculate through the penile meatus.[5]

In both sexes, it is clear that orgasm is a systemic physiological experience. Immediately before orgasm, the heart rate rises (20–80 beats/minute) as does the blood pressure (25–120 mm Hg systolic and 25–50 mm Hg diastolic).[6] Hyperventilation of up to 40 breaths a minute and contractions of foot muscles may also occur. As best as can be ascertained, orgasm feels comparable to both sexes. Orgasms vary in intensity; the more intense ones are felt body-wide and may be immediately followed by a brief sleep. Calm follows orgasm whether or not sleep ensues. Pelvic congestion is reversed. Men enter their refractory period, during which they are unresponsive to further tactile and erotic stimulation. The absence of a comparable refractory period in women provides some with the opportunity to realize multiple orgasms. Masters and Johnson labeled the post orgasm physiological events the *resolution phase* of sexual excitement.

SEXUAL SATISFACTION

When the three dimensions of sexual identity—gender, orientation, intention—and the three dimensions of sexual function—desire, arousal, and orgasm—are added together, the "anatomy" of our sexual selves is seen to have six components. These components will occupy us for the remainder of this book. But, there is another psychosocial matter that has confused clinicians and researchers alike: *satisfaction*. Sexual satisfaction, the seventh dimension of sexual "anatomy," should not be confused with the pleasure of orgasm.

Not only do we have a distinct sexual identity and a body that transports us from desire to calming orgasm, but we also invariably reflect on the comfort and ease with which we conduct our sexual lives and the behavior of our partners. These reflections are part of our capacity to integrate our sexual lives with our nonsexual relationship and our notions about what life should hold for us. People are often satisfied with sexually dysfunctional lives. The explanation may be: they do not know it might be considerably better; they are generally accepting people; or they weigh other factors in their lives as far more important. Similarly, people are often deeply unsatisfied with their sexual lives, although they have no sexual dysfunction. The explanation may be: they no longer like or respect their partner; their sexual identity needs are not met by their partner; or they think other people are having more excitement and fun.

Sometimes it seems that the sole reason for the existence of sexual satisfaction is to confound sexologic research. It is a constant reminder that objective assessment of human sexuality does not entirely capture the perception of sexual life. Sexual life, however it is realized in the bedroom, has highly individual meanings for people.

AN OUTLINE OF THE MAJOR PATHOLOGIES BROUGHT TO CLINICIANS

I. SEXUAL IDENTITY PROBLEMS
  A. Gender
    1. Gender identity disorder of childhood
    2. Transvestism
    3. Transsexualism

      4. Gender confusion
      5. Low self-esteem based on gender identity and role inadequacy
   B. Orientation
      1. Confusion
      2. Self-hatred on the basis of homosexuality
      3. Pedophilia
   C. Intention
      1. Single paraphilias
         a. Sadism
         b. Masochism
         c. Voyeurism
         d. Exhibitionism
         e. Pedophilia (see Orientation)
         f. Fetishism
      2. Multiple paraphilias
      3. Sexual compulsivity
         a. Seduction of partners
         b. Masturbation
II. SEXUAL DYSFUNCTIONS
   A. Desire disorders
      1. Absence or low level of drive
      2. Drive without motivation for partner
      3. Incompatible levels of desire with partner
      4. Mutual avoidance of sexual behavior
   B. Arousal disorders
      1. Lubrication problems with or without dyspareunia
      2. Vaginismus
      3. Erectile dysfunction
   C. Orgasm problems
      1. Anorgasmia
      2. Difficulty reaching orgasm
      3. Premature ejaculation
      4. Pleasureless orgasm
      5. Coital anorgasmia
III. LACK OF SATISFACTION
   A. Associated with one of the above problems
   B. Associated with no other sexual problem

SUMMARY

The pathologies of sexual life demonstrate to the clinician that there are seven individual components to every adult human being. These components (our sexual "anatomy") include three that comprise our sexual identity—gender, orientation, and intention; three that are essential to sexual function—desire, arousal, and orgasm; and one that integrates sexual experiences with the rest of our lives—sexual satisfaction. Sexual desire best illustrates the complexity of sexual selves. Desire is the end product of the integration of biological forces called *sexual drive*, psychological forces called *motive*, and social forces called *wish*.

REFERENCES

1. Kinsey AC, Pomeroy WB, Martin CE: *Sexual Behavior in the Human Male*. Philadelphia, WB Saunders, 1948.
2. Kaplan HS: *Disorders of Sexual Desire*. New York, Brunner/Mazel, 1979.
3. Swaab, DF, Fliers E: A sexually dimorphic nucleus in the human brain. *Science,* 1985; 228:1112–1115.
4. Levin RJ, Wagner G: Orgasm in women in the laboratory—quantification studies on duration, intensity, latency, and vaginal blood flow. *Archives of Sexual Behavior,* 1985; 14:439–450.
5. Masters WH, Johnson V: *Human Sexual Response*. Boston, Little, Brown, 1966.
6. Littler WA, Honour AJ, Sleight P: Direct arterial pressure, heart rate, and electrocardiogram during coitus. *Journal of Reproduction and Fertility,* 1974; 40:321–331.

CHAPTER 4

Psychological and Sexual Intimacy

The key to an emotionally rich life is the ability to establish and maintain psychological intimacy. Psychological intimacy enables relationships to form, motivates sexual behavior, and soothes the soul.

Psychological intimacy is an important ingredient of lovemaking, psychotherapy, and a few other matters of considerable relevance to mental health professionals. It is a vital, although subtle, enabler of sexual expression. This fact places psychological intimacy close to the heart of two of the five general forces that shape sexual expression: individual psychology and the quality of a couple's nonsexual relationship. When we are able to understand how psychological intimacy bridges these two forces, we will be closer to a practical clinical knowledge of what augments and limits sexual function for most people.

"THEY WERE INTIMATE"

In the past, the meaning of sentences like "they were intimate" confused me; now they amuse me. Here is why. The word *intimacy* has subtle connotations which imply contact with our innermost selves. "Intimate" and "intimacy" are unclear about whether these innermost touches are physical, psychological, or both. The word *intimacy* conjures up notions of familiarity, understanding, affection, and privacy. In doing so, it immediately draws us close to powerful ideas involving appropriateness or politeness.

Politeness, the rarely stated rules for proper social conduct that protect our privacy, often requires that innermost touches of any kind remain unspecified. The word *intimacy* does nicely when one wants to delicately refer to, but not name, breast or genital caressing or intercourse. The same word is used to convey an emotional or psychological closeness having nothing to do with sexual behavior. Adding to this ambiguity of usage is the possibility that female listeners tend to supply an emotional meaning to the term while male listeners tend to impose a sexual one.

Sexual intimacy holds a seemingly endless fascination for both sexes. Learning about it, however, is limited by oppressive attitudes toward discussing it. As a result, many people have never engaged in a calm, informed discussion about sexual life. Although sexual intimacy plays an important role in our lives, it pales in importance when compared with psychological intimacy. Yet, curiously, the nature of psychological intimacy remains uncertain to us, despite our frequent attempts to describe its relevance to our lives.

THE SIGNIFICANCE OF PSYCHOLOGICAL INTIMACY

Psychological intimacy is an important ingredient of high-quality human relationships. It is relevant to professional and nonprofessional relationships alike. I consider psychological intimacy to be a requirement for an emotionally rich life. Its significance derives from five of its capacities. Psychological intimacy causes: (1) important relationships to form; (2) motivation for sexual expression; (3) long-term quieting of the inner self; (4) a transient elusive state of grace that promises happiness; and (5) a multitude of complaints when it disappears.

Mental health professionals often act as though these capacities are not generally known. This is peculiar. Many clinicians recognize that psychological intimacy is the part of their daily lives that makes their work a pleasant refuge from ordinary nonclinical life. But beyond such privately expressed statements, little is now written about it in professional literature. Empathy,[1] intuition, introspection, identification, self-objects,[2] countertransference, transference, and intersubjective processes[3] all get professional attention, but not intimacy. I believe this is because intimacy, although basic to these intellectual concepts, has not been legitimized as a professional concept. When Eric Erikson introduced it many decades ago,[4] it was a professional concern. In recent decades, however, writings about it have almost exclusively been found in lay magazine articles and self-help books. These popular pieces encourage strategies for capturing or recapturing psychological intimacy; they are not concerned, as we are, with deciding what intimacy actually is and exactly how it is elicited.

It is rarely suggested in our professional literature that the diverse problems that mental health professionals treat may, at least in part, be due to the lack of psychological intimacy in the most important relationships of our patients' lives. Psychological intimacy has enormous significance for the conduct of psychotherapy in general, and for therapy of sexual difficulties in particular. It can best be appreciated in jargon-free language.

THE FIRST STEP TO PSYCHOLOGICAL INTIMACY

Psychological intimacy begins with one person's ability to share her or his inner experiences with another. This deceptively simple capacity actually rests upon several separate abilities: (1) the capacity to know what one feels and thinks; (2) the willingness to say it to another; and (3) the skills to express the feelings and the ideas with words. These abilities are specified separately because the chance of establishing and maintaining psychological intimacy is limited by the incapacity of any of them.

Some people do not recognize what they feel, even when their feelings are intense. The best they can do is to say that they are "upset" before or after they behave in some problematic manner. Others do not trust anyone enough to share their inner experiences. Still others are limited by their language skills; they know what they are experiencing but they cannot explain it.*

The crucial first step toward psychological intimacy begins when one person shares something from within the private self with another. It need not be elegantly said, lofty in its content, or unusual in any way; it just needs to be from the inner experience of the self—from the *soul*.†

Intimacy Requires Two

Even though we sometimes speak of a person knowing herself or himself intimately, psychological intimacy requires at least two people. Individuals differ widely in their ability to quickly know what they feel and to label it with exact words, such as anger, envy, sexual desire, ambition, or

---

*The first and third of these characteristics are now referred to as *alexithymia* in psychiatric circles.[5] This medical term derived from the Greek suggests that not knowing or not being able to speak about inner experience is a disorder. Alexithymia is described as a disturbance in communicative style with reduced symbolic thinking, inner attitudes, feelings, wishes, and drives that are not revealed; thinking is literal, utilitarian, and concerned with the minutiae of external events; there are few dreams; a paucity of fantasies; and trouble in distinguishing feelings from bodily sensations. This disorder is reputed to be more common in males, but cynicism or, at the very least, skepticism may be called for here: alexithymia may have medicalized the essence of culturally determined male gender role behavior.

†Sometimes I like to refer to the inner self as the *soul* in order to allude to the aspects of personal experience that cannot be grasped by technical terms, such as ego or personality. Of these many aspects, the most relevant to this discussion is love. The word *soul* is important to our experience of loving; after all, we often happily speak of our lovers as "soulmates." The word is a dangerous one in clinical work, however, because it carries a frequently misunderstood religious connotation.

guilt. When they can do this, they remain informed about the state of their inner selves. This highly sought-after state of knowing about and owning one's affects leads many people to spend untold time, money, and energy in various forms of psychotherapy. Knowing about all of our feelings, conflicts, and motives is not easy. The universality of this difficulty can be seen in the major concepts that sprang from psychoanalysis during the early part of the twentieth century. These words, once the brilliant discoveries of mental science, now are part of everyday language: *defenses, neuroses, resistance,* and *unconscious.* Each refers to another aspect of the obstacles that make overcoming our alienation from our inner selves arduous.

Although some people are so attuned to their external world that they pay relatively little attention to their inner experiences, others occupy the opposite end of this spectrum: they are so constantly oriented to their souls that they have trouble paying much attention to anything outside of themselves. For each of us, the ability to pay attention to our inner selves and the world around us is changeable. Our basic ability to know ourselves, however, usually fluctuates around the position we occupy on the self-aware versus world-aware spectrum.

It is tempting to refer to being intimate with ourselves because our relationship to ourselves sometimes feels as though we are two people: one who interacts with the world of people and tasks, and one who privately feels, thinks, and senses. Intimacy with the self is only a metaphor; self-awareness is not a substitute for psychological intimacy. At least two people are required for this state.

The ability to know what is going on within the self and, ultimately, to understand the many paradoxes and contradictions which are inherent in each of us is a reasonable predictor of the ability to enter into an intimate relationship with another person. The capacity for psychological intimacy is a bridge that links individual psychology to relationship capacity. Those who are terrified to know themselves may become frightened by the possibilities of real psychological intimacy. Genuine psychological intimacy begins with self-awareness, but is something different from it.

THE SECOND STEP TO PSYCHOLOGICAL INTIMACY

For intimacy to occur, one has to tell another person about the self and the other person has to respond in a manner that conveys (1) a noncritical acceptance of what is being said; (2) an awareness of the importance of the moment to the speaker; and (3) a grasp of what is being said. It also helps a great deal if the listener feels that it is a privilege to hear what the speaker has to say. The ideal condition for intimacy occurs when both the speaker and the listener sense the importance of the moment.

When a listener judges what is being said negatively by saying, "You shouldn't feel that way!" or does not acknowledge the significance of what is being said by impatiently remarking, "Can't this wait? Don't you see how busy I am?" or listens but misses the point of the speaker's words, intimacy will not occur.

General Obstacles

Many subtleties have to be in place for psychological intimacy to occur and recur. In separate ways, the speaker and the listener can each ensure that it does not take place. The speaker's lack of self-awareness, or unwillingness to share, or inability to express what is felt and the listener's criticism or ill-presented disagreement, or inability to perceive the meaning of the conversation to the speaker, or failure to grasp the speaker's point can rapidly end any hope of attaining or reestablishing this state of grace.

THE DEFINITION OF PSYCHOLOGICAL INTIMACY

Let us say that the listener responds correctly. What is the intimacy that will occur? What is the definition of psychological intimacy? Psychological intimacy is a simultaneous two-person combination of solace and pleasure. The solace of the speaker results from sharing the inner self, being listened to with interest, and being understood. The pleasure of the listener results from hearing about the speaker's inner experiences.

One-Sided and Two-Sided Intimacy

Intimacy has two basic forms. If the conversation continues with the speaker speaking and the listener listening, it is *one-sided*. But if they switch roles, the intimacy is *two-sided*. One-sided psychological intimacies are common between children and their parents, patients and health care professionals, clients and lawyers or accountants, and advice-seekers and clergy. Two-sided intimacies are the basis of friendships, love relationships, and are the best day-in-and-day-out aphrodisiacs ever discovered. Professional intimacies that begin as one-sided and become two-sided are often the forerunner to sexual exploitation of persons seeking help.

Within these two basic forms of psychological intimacy, there are countless degrees of self-disclosure and nuances of attention and understanding. No two intimacies are quite alike; each relationship is uniquely rich or poor in its possibilities. Persons who have seen two therapists often are aware that each professional, although helpful, makes an important contribution to the different intimate atmosphere that occurs.

IMMEDIATE AND SHORT-TERM CONSEQUENCES OF PSYCHOLOGICAL INTIMACY

The Visible Bond

On the way to the solace of being understood, and on the way to the pleasure and privilege of hearing another person's inner self, powerful emotions can be generated in the listener and the speaker, especially the speaker. Most outside observers can recognize that sharing the soul with a person who receives it well creates a bond between the speaker and the listener. Thereafter, each regards the other differently. The two people are together in a new way: They glance at each other differently; touch each other differently; laugh together differently; and can continue to discuss readily other aspects of their private selves.

The Internalization of the Other

Yet much more occurs within the two people than can be observed from outside of them. Within both the speaker and the listener, there is a feeling of attachment, a loss of the usual social indifference, a vision of the person as special. The emotional power of these intimate conversations can be enormous. The listener becomes internalized within the speaker and, to some extent, the speaker becomes internalized in the listener. Internalization has predictable qualitative consequences, whose intensity varies from relationship to relationship: for example, (1) imagining the person when she or he is not present; (2) inventing conversations with the person; (3) preoccupation with the person's physical attributes; (4) anticipation of the next opportunity to be together; and (5) thoughts about that person as a sex partner.

Transference/Countertransference

When psychological intimacy occurs, we begin to weave the person into our selves. Our new intimate partner is not only reacted to as a unique individual, she or he stimulates thoughts, feelings, and worries that we previously experienced in relationship to others. We take advantage of this process in some forms of psychotherapy by trying to teach patients how to use their preoccupations with us in order to learn about their past. Sometimes this therapeutic focus helps a person to "peel off" the transference to other people currently in their lives so that they can react to them on their own merits rather than in terms of how someone else treated them in the past.

But, we clinicians are human, and the processes that we study in our patients are transpiring in ourselves. Therapists also weave the patient into some of their psychic lives. Typically, this is to a far lesser degree than the patient's transference. The major point, however, is that psychological intimacy is an effective trigger for both transference and countertransference, and, therefore, it is a topic that mental health professionals must think about clearly.

Erotization of the Other

The amount of time required to imagine the person as a sex partner—that is, the speed of the erotization provoked by intimacy—is modified by at least six factors: age; sex; sexual orientation; social status; purpose in talking together; and the nature of other emotional commitments. If the pair consists of a comparably aged, socially eligible heterosexual man and woman, the erotization triggered by sharing of some aspects of their souls can occur with lightning speed—in both of them. Similarly, for a homosexual pair of men or women, erotization can occur in a flash. The stimulation of the erotic imagination may never occur, may take a long time to occur, or may occur only in a fleeting disguised way depending on how these six factors line up. The formation of a bond between two people, however, and the personal, deeply private responses to that bond are what is triggered by the intimacy.

Relationships among people of the same sex are valued in part because they afford an opportunity to share the self without the burden of erotization. Orientation guides erotization responses, but it does not absolutely prevent them.

The Privacy/Secrecy of Erotization

The specific emotional experiences that occur as a result of intimate conversations are usually guarded with extreme care—so much so that when these mental events happen to some people, they worry they are losing their minds. The primary teaching that culture provides us about these responses is that they are nothing to worry about if we are falling in love. The process is qualitatively similar with friendship, however. Some same- and opposite-sex friendships end abruptly without a satisfying explanation because one person cannot tolerate the excitement it creates. Some individuals may worry that the relationship is "homosexual" or could lead to future sexual behavior. These worried individuals need to know that all psychological intimacy has at least a tendency to provoke an eroticization of the person with whom it is shared.

IMPLICATIONS FOR TRAINING

When a therapist–patient team studies the mental processes of a patient in a psychodynamic psychotherapy, each participant should expect that the patient's erotization responses or defenses against them will be part of the patient's growth process. Most patients who are conscious of their erotization never mention it directly. Many therapists find their own reasons for not exploring this universal byproduct of psychological intimacy. A collusion of silence, of course, does not mean that erotization is not occurring.

With or without direct attention to the erotic concomitants of psychotherapy, the significance of psychological intimacy for the psychotherapist is that the ingredients that engender intimacy are the same ingredients that promote psychological growth in relationships between parent and child, lovers, therapist and one patient, or a therapist and a couple.[6] Clinicians are well positioned to realize that psychological intimacy often reveals the person's struggle to love and to be loved, regardless of where it takes place.

Most therapists have an opportunity to experience erotic transference and countertransference during their first year of work as a psychotherapist. Many trainees never discuss these feelings in supervision. Those who do, however, value their supervision more highly because of the intimacy with the supervisor that results and what they learn about their own and the patient's life.

The erotic responses to the intimacy of psychotherapy vary with the gender and the orientation of the patient and the therapist. Among heterosexual patients, these responses are most apparent with women patients and male therapists, but they are not rare between male patients and female therapists. Therapists in training benefit from a frank direct discussion of these issues and often find grateful relief in their opportunities to describe previous and current situations that have concerned them. Same-sex patients who are erotically preoccupied with their heterosexual therapists can be especially disconcerting for the beginning therapist because homoerotic responses to the patient may be self-diagnosed as meaning that the therapist is gay. This confronts the therapist with his or her own bierotic potentiality and lack of understanding of homosexual identity. Eventually, such personal responses will not be shocking or surprising.

Homosexual therapists may have an additional burden to bear when a same-sexed patient is erotically stimulated by them. It is considerably more difficult to bring this transference and its less intense countertransference to a supervisor because it carries with it the revelation of one's orientation, which may not be a safe thing to do in every training setting.

A small percentage of therapists become sexually involved with some of their patients during their professional lifetimes.[7] Most of these are men.* Most, but not all, involve women patients. Every mental health discipline is clear that such behavior always exceeds the ethical boundaries of the professional role. Every discipline holds the therapist responsible for this behavior regardless of the intensity of the patient's erotic transference. Some authors have wondered how much of such problematic behavior may be related to never having processed erotic transference and counter-transference with a supervisor.[8] If this is correct, pedagogical failure to discuss this topic more openly may be a great disservice to the community.

THE LONG-TERM EFFECTS OF PSYCHOLOGICAL INTIMACY

Continued sharing of the soul by the speaker and listener in a two-sided manner is necessary if psychological intimacy is to be maintained and each is to continue to feel enriched by the attachment. This process of attaining and reattaining psychological intimacy soothes the soul. It allows people to be seen, known, accepted, understood, and treated with uniqueness. When these effects are realized, both people feel an inner peace that is often described by lay persons as "feeling secure" and by mental health professionals as greater stability, self-cohesion, and self-esteem, or improved ego function.[9] When these effects are absent at critical moments in a relationship or generally absent chronically, the opposite inner experiences may result.

In psychotherapy literature, the absence of intimacy is sometimes discussed as a specific failure of the empathic connection between parents and children, lovers, or spouses. In any of these pairs, immediate mental suffering results when the significant person fails to be interested in the other person's affects and their meanings. Some theorists consider that the parental failure to remain a good listener to a child's affect can provide a model for the origin of chronic emotional problems:[10] When the affect that was repudiated by the parent is experienced once again—for example, with a lover—its full conscious expression will be defended against. The affect, itself, becomes the source of conflict. What originally set up the defense is forgotten. The person is left with a disability in regard to that affect and the appreciation of its meanings. This is a technical psychodynamic way of saying that the consequences of failing to maintain intimacy can be highly destructive to the mental health of children and lovers.

---

*Likewise, a small percentage of supervisors become involved sexually with a trainee during supervision. The same forces that are triggered by psychological intimacy between therapist and patient occur in the minds of trainees and their valued supervisors as well.

THE RELATIONSHIP BETWEEN PSYCHOLOGICAL AND SEXUAL INTIMACY

Psychological intimacy does not usually lead to sexual behavior between people, but it can. Psychological intimacy lays the groundwork for people to become lovers. It enables them to make love again and again, and to shed their inhibitions during lovemaking so that they can eventually discover the limits of their sexual potential with one other.

Most people briefly realize at least a semblance of psychological intimacy when their relationship originally forms. But, quickly one of intimacy's basic characteristics becomes apparent: its positive psychological and sexual effects are relatively short-lived and so it must be recreated. This requires each partner to set aside time to reestablish it when the sense of unconnection or distance is felt by either of them. This can be a formidable problem for those who do not intuitively understand these ideas, cannot provide the speaking or listening requirements, are chronically overwhelmed by other demands, or who originally could manage only a one-sided or meager two-sided intimacy. As a result, the sexual potential of psychological intimacy does not get realized.

There is another more enigmatic obstacle that may appear in those who both understand, are generally capable of, and aspire to this state of grace. When the opportunity to attain psychological intimacy is present, individuals sometimes mysteriously become irritable or otherwise behave in a manner that makes emotional connection impossible. It is as though there is a powerful force within the person that fights the desire for intimate connection. This force may exasperate both the eager-for-intimacy partner and the person who sullies the opportunity.

Between the external demands of life, the limited capacities of people to recreate intimacy, and the occasional need to have emotional separateness from a partner, it is quite common for men and women to complain that there is insufficient intimacy in their lives. Two bypass strategies are frequently employed in order to attain the benefits of intimacy without the processes of speaking and listening: *mind reading* and *sexual behavior*.

Mind Reading

To some extent, most people are mind readers. Many spouses, for instance, are highly skilled at deducing or guessing what their partners are feeling and thinking from a glance. Mind reading, as therapists dealing with silent patients can testify, has four distinct limitations: (1) incorrect deductions are likely; (2) only a small fraction of another person's thoughts can be deduced; (3) the process soon becomes boring; and (4) inscrutability provokes abandoning the aspiration for psychological and physical closeness.

Sexual Behavior

To recreate emotional closeness, many people, especially men, generally have more faith in the power of sexual behavior than in mind reading. This point of view is understandable, although far from infallible. After all, sometimes even a kiss, let alone breast or genital contact, changes a relationship and creates a nonverbal yet profound sense of knowing the other person. Busy people with dwindling time and energy during their day easily come to rely on sexual interaction to recreate closeness. It works, but not invariably. It also does not work as a long-term strategy as many people have assumed. One of its dangers is that one person may think it is working while the other is certain that it is not. Such a couple usually has little capacity to talk about their differing reactions to their sexual behavior. It continues until the illusion is shattered: one person becomes recognizably sexually dysfunctional or unmistakably angry.

Sex as a substitute for psychological intimacy probably works best during early adulthood, but as most men and women age into midlife, they need better psychological conditions to make love in a way that reliably delivers both physical and psychological satisfaction. Better psychological conditions are brought about by the establishment and reestablishment of this two-person interaction that simultaneously creates solace and pleasure.

As we shall see in the next chapter, psychological intimacy is not the universal requirement for sexual arousal. For some people, in fact, psychological intimacy precludes sexual desire and makes sexual behavior difficult.

SUMMARY

Psychological intimacy begins in a moment of time between two people, a speaker and a listener. Depending on how well they fulfill these roles, each may be deeply comforted: the speaker can know the gratification of being understood; the listener can relish being granted private information. Such moments, particularly when long lasting or repeated, change how the speaker and listener regard one another and behave together. In doing so, each of their souls may be calmed.

Whether it occurs between a parent and child, homosexual lovers, a therapist and a patient, two people on a date, or husband and wife, psychological intimacy's greatest potential is its capacity to enhance psychological functioning. It creates a safe, trusting holding environment that harkens back to the best of parent–child relationships. If two people can recurrently establish psychological intimacy with ease, they often think of their relationship in loving terms, regardless of whether they have a sexual relationship. Great friendships are this way.

The services of mental health clinicians begin with high quality listening. We should not be surprised when the one-sided psychological intimacy that we provide creates erotic feelings in the patient, even if these feelings are never directly mentioned. Neither should we be surprised when such feelings occur in us.

REFERENCES

1. Basch MF: Empathic understanding: A review of the concept and some theoretical considerations. *Journal of American Psychoanalytic Association,* 1983; 31:101–126.
2. Ornstein PH, Ornstein A: Clinical understanding and explaining: The empathic vantage point, in Goldberg A (ed), *Progress in Self-Psychology.* New York, Guilford Press, 1985.
3. Stolorow R, Brandshaft B, Atwood G: *Psychoanalytic Treatment: An intersubjective approach.* Hillsdale, NJ. Analytic Press, 1987.
4. Erikson, EH: *Childhood and Society.* New York, Norton, 1950.
5. Taylor GJ: Alexithymia: Concept, measurement, and implications for treatment. *American Journal of Psychiatry,* 1984; 41(6):725–732.
6. Lear J: *Love in Its Place in Nature.* New York, Farrar, Strauss, & Giroux, 1991.
7. Gartrell N, Olarte S, Feldstein M, Localio JB: Psychiatrist-patient sexual contact: Results of a national survey. I: Prevalence. *American Journal of Psychiatry,* 1986; 143(9):1126–1131.
8. Gabbard GO (ed): *Sexual Exploitation in Professional Relationships.* Washington, D.C., American Psychiatric Press, 1989.
9. Frayn DH: Intersubjective processes in psychotherapy. *Canadian Journal of Psychiatry,* 1990; 35(5): 434–438.
10. Stolorow R, Brandshaft B: Developmental failure and psychic conflict. *Psychoanalytic Psychology,* 1987; 4:241–253.

CHAPTER 5

The Paradoxes of Sexual Desire

Drive, motive, wish, lust, affection, love, and maturity are the elements contained within the dramas of sexual desire. Long-term observation of the fluctuating alignment of these ingredients may transform the clinician into a student of love.

Sexual desire, the force that propels people toward physical intimacies, became the object of specific psychiatric study during the late 1970s when sex therapists realized that a large percentage of patients with arousal problems had little interest in behaving sexually.[1] They conceived of the diagnosis "hypoactive sexual desire" to account for the limited effectiveness of therapy with these men and women. Very quickly, clinicians recognized that sexual desire disorders were widespread and important. Desire problems came of age in 1983 when the *Diagnostic and Statistical Manual of Mental Disorders* (DSM-III) included "inhibited sexual desire" in its list of mental disorders for the first time.

This formal recognition also kindled interest in normal sexual desire. Workers in this area soon came to appreciate the many meaningful roles played by sexual desire during the life cycle. Sexual desire

1. Contributes to the evolution of sexual identity
2. Creates an adolescent drama whose resolution may yield acceptance of the legitimacy of bodily pleasures
3. Is integral to the formation of sexual relationships
4. Is a force to be managed in many nonsexual relationships
5. Enables procreation
6. Is a barometer of relationship vitality
7. Provides for the nurturance of both partners
8. Enables a richer understanding of the lives of others

This list is helpful in identifying the toll that significant desire problems take on a person's and a couple's life.

THE EPIDEMIOLOGICAL PARADOX

Epidemiology is the medical science that studies the causes and effects of diseases in population groups. It often begins its work with definitions of prevalence, the extent of the disease currently in a population, and incidence, the number of new cases per time period in a population. These basic questions depend upon having concepts of "How much desire is normal?" "How little is pathological?" and "How much represents a sickness?" Currently, such questions can be answered only arbitrarily. The prevalence and incidence of desire problems—both too little and too much—are uncertain. This is not surprising since there is a conspicuous absence of epidemiological knowledge about these parameters for most sexual dysfunctions.[2]

Since the pioneering studies published in 1948 and 1952 of Kinsey and his colleagues, most attempts to ascertain prevalence have used small samples from medical clinics or surveys in popular magazines.[3] Although such data may seem to be helpful, they usually reflect more about the medical clinic than the prevalence of sexual dysfunction in the community in which the clinic is located. An opportunity to study the prevalence of sexual dysfunction with careful population-based methods was bypassed when the prevalence data for the major mental disorders in five United States communities were gathered without including questions about sexual life.[4]

In the absence of community-based data, statements are often made by clinicians about the subject. These statements arise from their experience in working in a specific setting and in seeing an unclearly characterized slice of the population who are drawn to the setting by economic conditions, referral patterns, marketing, and geography. Whether such statements are made after a careful numerical review of the data or are simply stated impressionistically, they do not reliably reflect the actual prevalence of sexual problems in the population. They may, however, reflect the experiences of clinicians. Here is my experience:

Currently, among women and couples who seek help for sexual dysfunction problems, the most common complaint is some problem with sexual desire.[5] These problems can have an individual focus, such as absent, too low, or excessive desire; or a two-person focus, such as an incompatible pattern of desire. The desire problem may have always been present or may have developed suddenly or inconspicuously. Desire problems frequently hide behind other dysfunctions, such as erectile dysfunction and anorgasmia, and can be present when patients seek assistance for problems that are not sexual in focus. Whatever the actual prevalence and incidence of desire problems may be, it is important for clinicians to be familiar with their intricacies.

WHAT IS SEXUAL DESIRE?

No one is certain as to what sexual desire actually is. During the early part of this c   nt to assume that, like aggression, sexual   c biologically based instincts.
The manifes   erred to as *libido*. Libido was
understood t   : of human beings. As a basic
life force, libi   alth, repressed into neurosis,
and acted ou   few people speak of psychological life sii   of instincts and their derivatives. Psycho   e libido theory, has gone far
beyond its ea   orks. Other systems of think-
ing about mental life have generated hypotheses about other forces that shape personality development—for instance, cognitions, social learning, behavioral conditioning, and relationships.

When clinicians think about the nature of sexual desire, their hypotheses are usually consistent with the tenets of their preferred theory of mental functioning. When researchers deal with the subject, they are more interested in data than in ideology. Researchers' underlying concepts about the nature of sexual desire sometimes can be divined from the questions they ask of their subjects. Typically, these questions focus on: sexual fantasies; sexual dreams; initiation of self-stimulation to orgasm; initiation of sexual behavior with a partner; receptivity to sexual behavior; genital sensations; and heightened responsivity to erotic cues in the environment. Therefore, sexual desire may be whatever produces these subjective and behavioral changes.

A Working Definition

My formal definition of sexual desire is the psychobiologic energy that precedes and accompanies arousal and that tends to create sexual behavior. Sexual desire is a confusing concept because it consists of three inconstant elements; a biological element called *drive*; a psychological element called *motive*; and a social element called *wish*. These elements are much clearer conceptually than they are operationally. It is not a simple matter to go from the concept of desire to the questions that clearly separate drive, motivation, and wish, even though clinical judgments sometimes require it.

SEXUAL DRIVE: THE BIOLOGIC ASPECT OF SEXUAL DESIRE

Unfortunately, in my definition, the term *energy* is not a much more advanced concept than instinct. The energy of sexual desire is probably the result of activation of a neural network that is orchestrated by a series of neurotransmitters—dopamine, serotonin, and gamma-aminobutyric acid (GABA). In laboratory animals, from rats to primates, this network is called the *sexual drive center*. It has been located in the anterior-medial preoptic area of the hypothalamus and has been found to have extensive connections to the limbic system. Many investigations support this new concept. Anatomic destruction of the area stops the sexual behaviors of animals. Pharmacologic treatment with neurotransmitter agonists increases sexual behaviors while antagonists block them.[6,7]

The sexual drive center has been localized to the same area in humans, where, in preliminary studies, it was found to be twice as big in adult males than in adult females. A strong suggestion of a decline of the size of these hypothalamic nuclei with advancing age exists.

Clinicians are not interested in the basic anatomy and physiology of sexual drive for background knowledge alone. We have frequent practical concerns about its biological suppression by medications and its psychological suppression by unpleasant affects.

Several classes of drugs have been implicated in causing decreased sexual interest, especially at high dosages, including antihypertensives, antipsychotics, anticonvulsants, antidepressants, antiandrogens, and substances that increase estrogen levels, such as digitalis and spironolactone.[8] Clinical judgments may be difficult because every drug in these categories does not have the same impact on drive—for instance, a beta blocking agent may be more destructive to drive manifestations than an angiotensin-converting enzyme (ACE) inhibitor. In addition, patients have individual responses to medications that are not well understood—a beta blocker does not suppress every person's drive.

Clinical work would be simpler if drive were an autonomous mental force that remained unaffected by social and psychological circumstances. But the perception of drive may be dampened by: environments that encourage children not to think about such evils (such conditioning seems to work better with girls than with boys); despair or any of its related persistent depressive states; relationships that apparently hold no hope for sexual expression; and the decision to seek revenge on a partner by refusing to engage in sexual behavior. This leaves clinicians uncomfortable with a quick judgment that if sexual drive manifestations are low or absent, something is biologically amiss. The biology of drive may, in fact, be amiss, but one can be easily fooled.

Sexual drive is known to be dependent on the presence of a critical level of testosterone. In males this level—300–800 ng/dL—is 10 to 15 times higher than in females. Testosterone seems to be necessary for the creation of erotic fantasy, but not for erections in response to visual sexual stimulation. Testosterone can restore sexual drive to most recently hypogonadal men. Women complaining of the absence of sexual drive do not usually have subnormal testosterone levels and do not respond to testosterone replacement. The one important possible exception to this is in young surgically menopausal women.[9]

As science advances in this area, more specific mechanisms of action of testosterone and medications may be defined. There probably are multiple mechanisms whereby drugs impair sexual drive including those that involve testosterone and those that do not. A valid biological measurement that reflects drive levels would help immensely. It is particularly difficult to recognize psychologically suppressed drive in older people, who can be too quickly dismissed as having an age-related organic loss of drive.

SEXUAL MOTIVE: THE PSYCHOLOGICAL ASPECT OF SEXUAL DESIRE

Over the course of the life cycle, particularly in middle and older ages when the frequency and intensity of sexual drive manifestations lessen, sexual motive is the primary determinant of when and if partner sexual behavior occurs. Motive is manifested by a willingness to behave sexually. This willingness involves either initiation, receptivity, or both. Although initiation is stereotypically thought of as a male characteristic and receptivity as a female characteristic, each person, regardless of gender, has moments of direct and subtle initiation and receptivity.

Clinical work with patients who have sexual drive but are motivated to avoid sexual behavior with their partners has produced an understanding of three major influences on the motivational component of sexual desire. Although these can be simply stated, their clinical recognition can be difficult:

1. Regard for the partner
2. Gratification of sexual identity needs
3. Negative transference

The most clinically obvious determinant of motive is how the person privately regards the partner. Anger over unresolved nonsexual issues, disappointments with the partner's habitual behavioral style, and disrespect over the lack of honesty or integrity, for example, can make sexual behaviors unpalatable. A motive to behave sexually can be quickly replaced with an overriding motive to avoid physical intimacy when the partner is perceived to be unworthy in some way. For example, a woman beginning therapy for her longstanding vaginismus discovers her husband's infidelities. "Now, making love is the *last* thing I want to do!"

The second and more clinically subtle contributor to motive is sexual identity. Sexual identity of the individual may be a secret from the partner or from oneself. Many enigmatic motives to avoid sex with partners yield to the realization that the avoidant person prefers a role in which a different gender can be personally assumed, the sex of the partner would be different, or an unusual sexual behavior would occur. These can be summarized by saying that the motive to behave sexually considerably weakens when some aspect of the individual's subjective sexual identity needs are not met by the partner. In these clinical situations, drive usually acts in opposition to motive, and partner sexual behavior becomes less frequent and intense or disappears. The inability to know about unmet sexual identity needs or to share it with the partner creates the mystery that leads to the formal diagnosis of a sexual desire disorder. If the clinician fails to inquire about sexual identity, the etiology will be considered idiopathic. But if a history of each component of identity is carefully taken, the clinician can help the person or couple deal more directly with the tangible issues that have to be faced.

The third, and most subtle, contributor to motive is an anxious, untrusting, or hostile transference. A sexual partner is not just a person with a self-defined identity and real characteristics. A partner is also unconsciously defined by the individual in terms that better fit parents or past lovers. The key concept here is unconscious because, as best as can be clinically determined, past experiences can be completely forgotten yet can exert a powerful influence. Forgotten sexual abuse at the hands of a trusted adult in the family, for example, has the potential to paralyze the person's motive to behave sexually with a loved partner. The memory of abuse may be partially reactivated during current sexual behavior. It is kept out of awareness by anxiety or the inability to relax long enough to sensually experience lovemaking. These patterns gradually create a motive to avoid participation in partner sexual behavior. Whatever drive is present is opposed by the motive to avoid the reexperiencing of the memories of past trauma. It is easier to avoid partner sexual behavior than to return to the past with its painful affects, conflicts, and meanings.

A similar scenario can account for inhibited sexual desire without actual sexual abuse. It has long been thought that parents who are consistently seductive, emotionally distant, or capricious in their interest in their children may leave their grown-up children anxious in their adult relationships.

Transference is not just a negative phenomenon. Past loving, trusting, caring relationships enable people to assume that their future lovers will be reasonable human beings who will not go out of their way to take advantage of or misuse them. Negative transferences are a reminder that victims of poor past relationships may not recover sexually even though the rest of their lives seem fine. When inhibited sexual desire is due to negative transferences, the clinician usually needs some time with the patient before this etiology can be perceived with conviction. As with the lack of respect for the partner and unmet sexual identity needs, however, if the clinician is not alert to the possibility or does not ask, the etiology may be missed.

Willingness to behave sexually seems to be the result of a person's capacity to synthesize sexual identity, current views of the partner's trustworthiness, and the influence of past relationships. These three factors explain much of the content of the psychotherapy of sexual motivation problems.

SEXUAL WISH: THE SOCIAL DIMENSION OF SEXUAL DESIRE

Historians, sociologists, philosophers, theologians, and anthropologists each remind clinicians that sexual life is influenced by forces that surround the individual and are more important than the details of the person's life. Some early Christian sects, for example, considered sex to be a demonic evil that had to be constantly fought against through repudiation of bodily desires and sensations. The "flesh" was evil. The legacy of these ideas about the darkness of sexual feelings goes far beyond the few individuals who managed to live ascetically in order to overcome their desire: they have lesser manifestations in many people who live during and after the time the ideas are in ascendancy.

All sexual behaviors occur within a social field that extends from the person to the couple, the community, the region, the nation, and time in history. These social influences mysteriously find their way to personal expectations about sexual behavior.

Sexual wishes or cognitions are readily confused with motives to behave sexually because they, too, can be emotionally powerful. Wishes, however, range in power from the trivial lies we tell ourselves about our sexual lives—"I want to have sexual intercourse three times a week"—to unfortunate matters of conscience that constrain sexual behavior for a lifetime—"Nice women do not enjoy sexual life for themselves; they provide for their husbands," or "Masturbation is a sin for which you will burn eternally in Hell." These ideas are acquired from the developing person's environment, but just because they each have a traceable pathway to a time in history or a subcultural tenet, does not mean that they can be simply eradicated from people's minds with education.

Chief among the personal expectations about sex that have an enormous hold on women and men are those that derive from the patriarchal organization of culture and that define roles on the basis of gender rather than on the basis of a person's interests and abilities. Patriarchal influences on sexual life can be seen in some couples who will only have intercourse in the missionary position because the man-on-top feels "normal" or in men who will stimulate women but will not passively receive any sensual attention because it is not "natural." To the extent that women's romanticism is culturally conditioned and reinforced, the patriarchal influence can be seen here as well. Romanticism may be partially a defense against personal recognition of bodily sensations and explicit fantasies of lovemaking—perhaps it is of social utility to "men" not to have women clearly aware of their bodily selves.

Clinicians are emotionally powerful authorities to people who are seeking their help. The patient–clinician relationship is a social interaction that provides for new ideas, novel-to-the-patient cognitions, that may eventually replace the older powerful ideas that have managed to constrain sexual expression.

Sexual desire is by its very nature paradoxical. Within the seeming homogeneity of sexual desire is an enormous potential for conflict. Few people can maintain the illusion of having no conflicts about their sexual desires. The paradoxes go beyond the desire's masquerade as a simple appetite and the opposing directions in which drive, motive, and wish may push the person. Often several different and conflicting motives and wishes coexist and possess enough power to completely mask the manifestations of sexual drive.

IS SEXUAL DESIRE ONLY EARLY AROUSAL?

Since the late 1970s, the standard teaching has been that sexual function could be divided into the separate physiological processes of desire, arousal, and orgasm. As clinical experience has increased with desire problems, however, two observations have challenged this axiom. First, desire is clearly much more than physiological drive. Second, arousal can stimulate desire as well as be produced by it.

Perhaps arousal is the first mental event in the sexual physiological sequence. This idea is given some credence by the intriguing idea that every person has an erotic script, a personally derived scenario, that is formed prior to or soon after puberty and that organizes sexual fantasy and behavior in a subtle way thereafter.[10] This is an idea that there is a basic, central erotic fantasy, a type of erotic template that is stimulated by both drive and environmental cues that fit the template.

The tripartite description of sexual desire has clinical utility, but it may be too limited to elucidate the psychology of robust, ordinary, or impaired sexual function. Other aspects of desire must be considered, beginning with lust.

LUST

Lust is not the same as desire, drive, arousal, or love. I reserve the word for the efficient, intense, subjective arousal provoked by imagery. For heterosexual men, this imagery usually, but not exclusively, is of relatively young women. Lust is stimulated by clothed or naked body parts and postures of women that suggest their desire to do the man's sexual bidding. It is important that little else about the woman be known—certainly not her psychological humanity. For a woman to provoke lust, she must be thought of as being a certain type[11]—nothing much more. Lust is provoked by sexual fantasy, films, reading material, or contacts with strangers. Each of these protects the man from his usual understanding of the complexity of male–female relationships and gratifies his curiosity about the privacy of women's bodies and behaviors. Lust requires simplicity, body parts, and the notion that the other person is aching to be sexually available. Probably the most common experiences with this quick efficient   . Men value their transient excitements w   strated by their pleasure in looking at wome

The   male homosexual lust except that the body   behaviors are male-centered. Lust is usuall   non, but heterosexual and homosexual w   ell.

Ado   body parts that are their favorites because   of pleasure and arousal. Women are capable of longing for simple, physical sex without the usual constraints of real relationships. Women can find media depictions of sexual behavior arousing. So-called female pornography, or sexually explicit imagery designed to appeal more specifically to heterosexual women, rests upon the same power of body imagery to provoke excitement, except that there often is a greater attempt to convey something about a relationship. It is not much different among lesbian women.

Lustful arousal can be so powerful, riveting, and enjoyable that it is possible to experience it without paying much attention to the psychological subtleties that allow it to emerge. But when attention is paid to heterosexual lust, it is usually possible to perceive a power differential between the man who is being excited and the woman whose body and posturing are the source of arousal. Such images are not universally exciting but they are quite commonly arousing. Men and women, but especially women, may eventually realize the inequality in these scenes and repudiate them as degrading to women and harmful to men in allowing them to assume an unearned power in heterosexual relationships devoid of attachment. The degradation and control of women in lustful images are the basis for the idea that lust contains a disguised element of aggression. Repudiated or not, containing aggression or not, it is striking how powerful such imagery can be for either sex and how these lust experiences may become a measuring devise to use when comparing subsequent partner experiences.

The specifics of lust vary according to sexual identity. Everyone, however, is capable of this intensely subjective powerful realization that imagery, not personhood, can sneak into the psyche and suddenly create sensations of arousal. Lust feels as though it is a combination of an intense drive and a strong motive to behave sexually. Its impressive power to overcome usual social inhibitions is probably the basis for the fact that many people consider its stimuli to be a social danger and a personal evil. Lust supports the idea that there is a central erotic script. When conditions of the script are met, minds respond with intense arousal. When these conditions are not met, the imagery quickly becomes boring. When the images that accompany the problems of excessive sexual desire are discussed in the chapter on paraphilia (Chapter 11), we will have an opportunity to further consider the psychology and ramifications of lust.

CASUAL AND COMMITTED AVENUES TO SEXUAL AROUSAL

Some of the mysteries of women and men who are diagnosed with inhibited sexual desire yield to another paradox of desire: it is difficult for some of these people to be sexually aroused with partners whom they love.

Most people who rely on lustful images for masturbation eventually turn to sexual relationships with real people and find that their mutual experiences are more enjoyable than self-stimulation with fantasy. As they progress to the complexity of heterosexual relationships, many of them take a long time to be able to initiate and sustain honest mutuality. In the meantime, casual sex, sexual intimacies without commitment, seduction, or sex with relative strangers can be highly arousing. Apparently, these relationships are the next step forward from the lustful imagery of masturbation. They must maintain some of the intensity of lust because they are admired and celebrated by culture throughout the ages especially in Don Juan themes. Of course, many people tire of this relationship style and are willing to trade fidelity for mutual commitment. This is the critical point in the life cycle; the developmental road forks into three directions: some individuals manifest symptoms of inhibited sexual desire; for others, sex loses some of its intensity; for others, sexual life begins in earnest.

Concepts of psychosexual maturity stress the necessity of integrating sexual excitement into a relationship with a partner for whom affection is the dominant feeling. Some otherwise enigmatic desire problems are a manifestation of the person's inability to experience sexual excitement with a person who is the object of their respect and affection. The sexual desire disorder disappears immediately when the person returns to casual or uncommitted relationships—that is, relationships closer to lustful scenes that have been imagined or remembered for years. Talking to these women and men may reveal that the central erotic fantasy is based on sex with relative strangers, or to uncommitted relationships. Their life experiences demonstrate a dramatic change from good to impaired sexual function when their lives depart too much from their longstanding fantasy.

Sigmund Freud explained this phenomenon in men as due to an unresolved Oedipal conflict. He pointed out that potency was often enhanced by the man's perception of his partner as inferior in some way—by social class, intelligence, vocation, family background, or power.[12] He thought that men mentally degraded their partners so as not to transfer their tender feelings about their mothers to their sexual partners.

Freud conceived of the Oedipal phase as the time of a boy's life when he was able to have deep affection for, and physical excitement over, his mother. His growing awareness that this ideal situation was untenable because of his powerful father led to the splitting apart of the affection and the sexual excitement. The affection stayed with his mother, while his sexual excitement was displaced outside the family. Much of adolescent sexual experimentation involved attempts to bring excitement and affection together in one person. Sexual maturity was attained when this was accomplished. Freud's 1914 formulation still has a strong appeal for explaining the phenomenon of women and men who are able to love and to have good sex, but not with the same person. Sometimes these people dramatically become sexually impaired when engagement or marriage occurs. The partner is perceived as "too good" to have sex with—that is, to be defiled by aggressive animalistic pleasures. This predicament is sometimes called the "madonna–whore complex."

The Paradox Continues

Even though many people spend most of their single lives trying to find a suitable committed relationship, they may prefer imagery of casual sex in the privacy of their subjective experiences. When they do reach "maturity" and can experience pleasurable arousal with a valued human being whose thoughts, feelings, and interests matter to them, they often joke about the "good old days" when sex was more intense and exciting. I am not certain whether all of this is explained by the Oedipal complex. What I do feel certain about is that some people lose their sexual vitality within committed relationships while others can only find it there. Society, through its mental health professionals, diagnoses the former people as having inhibited sexual desire, if they come to our clinical attention.

LOVE

Is it reasonable to consider the topic of love when trying to understand sexual desire? Love may be the ultimate context for comprehending the integration of sexual drive, motive, and wish. It is deeply embedded in our expectations that the vicissitudes of desire bear some relationships to our longings to love and be loved. Curiously, our aspirations to sustain a life in which we are a vital ingredient in another person's happiness have generally been of little direct interest to the mental health professions. Psychiatry has avoided the topic for most of this century, preferring to focus on disorders rather than on life processes. Perhaps for good reasons: the subject of love is endlessly subjective; human experience with it may be too individual to discern the principles governing its comings and goings, if indeed there are underlying principles; everyone has love stories to tell; and objective clinical science does not seem to have the tools to approach the magic of love. Psychiatric discussion of love have been written, but these writers have no monopoly on illuminating ideas about it. This vast subject belongs more properly to all of the humanities.

Our patients sometimes act as though we have answers to their personal struggles with love's mysteries. In the genius of retrospect, we may sometimes lose our humility by providing answers to the great question, "Why did I end up with this partner?" Our answers usually rest upon similarities to parents because many clinicians believe, on the basis of theory and elegant case examples, that all development involves a continuing working through of the family of origin issues, chief among which is the Oedipal complex. The matter of partner choice is a *great* question, but great questions should not be answered too quickly by formula; it robs the patient of the dignity of ongoing personal discovery and the answers, in fact, are often a gross oversimplification.

Psychotherapists are in a position of thinking about love from a vantage point that exceeds their personal lives simply because women and men in therapy talk all the time about their aspirations to love and be loved. From the vantage point of long-term psychotherapy, it often seems correct that concerns about loving and being loved are central in many patients' minds, regardless of their diagnoses.

Our knowledge about this important, overdetermined, affect-laden state is descriptive and speculative. Consider some of the redundant, imprecise language that is used to describe the wonders of adult attachment: falling in love, crush, infatuation, romantic love, passionate love, passionate romantic love, passion, limerance, tender love, affectionate love, true love, companionate love, and mature love. The first eight of these terms seem to be nearly synonymous for the emotional excitement of the beginnings of love, which some people experience at the start of their emotional attachment to another person. It is difficult to discuss falling in love without using the term *romantic love*, however, since romance is so celebrated in the culture.

Not everyone is patient with discussions of romance. Skepticism often greets these considerations. Skeptics consider romantic love to be unhealthy—a fantasy rather than reality, a cultural-based product, an artifact of human experience stimulated by the advertising and film industries, which is unworthy of serious attention. When a skeptic calls a person a "romantic," it is not usually a compliment. The concept of romantic love does not go away just because of skepticism, rationality, and science, however, and even skeptics long for its imagined fruits.

Falling in Love

Falling in love is usually described as an all-encompassing, intense, impermanent experience which ideally gives way to rich, deep, lasting, and fulfilling love but, instead, frequently ends in profound disappointment.[13,14]

Falling in love often feels as though it has happened to the person from something outside the self (hence, Cupid's arrow). People often use the verb *struck* to capture its beginnings. Psychologists, however, surmise that whether it occurs in youth, midlife, or old age, it typically is preceded by the need for change in one's life. The process is heavily dominated by fantasy and often contains a degree of suffering. The suffering may simply be the anticipation of not having the love requited. People who have fallen in love are preoccupied with the fantasies of opening themselves up to their lover. The joy of falling in love derives from the perception that this person seems destined to fulfill previously unmet longings. The pain of it derives from the vulnerability to rejection.

When people are in the midst of falling in love, their passion for their beloved reorganizes their lives. The loved person is idealized and is seen as a catalyst for the emergence of new improved elements in the personality. Early on, such love thrives on mystery, unavailability, and often the sense of transgression and danger.

Individuals in this state want to be with their beloved. They think and want to talk about their beloved a great deal. They so idealize their partner that they consider the person to be superior to others. They may even think they are having a unique experience that others could not possibly understand. Others, however, experience them as blinded to the real traits of their lover. Freud referred to this state of being in love as the only normal form of psychosis! Falling in love helps some people to realize the emptiness of their current lives. In the hope of finding more inner peace and happiness, this vibrant emotional state emboldens many people to make dramatic changes in the structure of their lives.

In the early stages of requited love, the new partners often cannot get enough of each other sexually. Frequently, they are amazed at the change in their levels of desire from their ordinary patterns. What seems to be happening was best described by Plato: two souls are finally being fused into one being; each soul has found its long-missing part. To use more formal psychiatric language, each person is remaking the self through new identifications with the other. This joyful state of (re)union sometimes enables a rapid and complete loss of sexual inhibition and an "incredible" sexual pleasure, which adds to the lovers' convictions that they have found their missing halves. Sexual bliss has not always been the expected consequence of reciprocated love. At some epochs, and today in some subcultures, sexual expression has been prohibited even among those who are "smitten" with each other.

The absence of such glorious intensity at the start of a relationship does not predict a loveless life. If the real fit between the two people continues to be as good as was originally imagined, the individuals move on to deal with other life issues and developmental tasks. A quieter affection, harmony, and mutual enhancement of self-esteem replace the passion of romantic love or appear even though passion did not mark the beginning.

When such passionate excitements do initially occur, they often end surprisingly fast. Some obstacle in the self, the other, or both is often discovered making the lover into something very far from what was imagined. Suddenly, the now disappointed person, laden with painful affects, wonders, " What did I ever see in him (her)?" "Why did I let this happen?" Some of these disappointed people find themselves in psychotherapy.

> Amy, aged 41, beautiful but unable to find an enduring relationship, previously had eight visits with me to discuss her recent absent sexual drive and avoidance of lovemaking. She quickly realized that she did not want to marry her rarely employed companion but was afraid to be without his doting attention. She soon made their relationship officially platonic and tried to believe me that her desire problem was related to her judgments about this man's character and her worries about her future with him.
>
> Most of her therapy focused on her devoted sacrificial relationship to her father in his business and the story of how he betrayed her by selling his business to an outsider without even discussing it with her.
>
> Six months later, she fell in love and had the best sex of her life. She throbbed with desire for him all the time. There was a serious problem, however. ["It is never easy with me."] He was married! Although he did not seem to care, she did. She had never dated a married man before, felt intensely guilty, and did not want to hurt his wife and children, whom she recently glimpsed together. As she was deciding what to do with the tension between her guilt and her incredible excitement, he made it easier by failing to deliver on his promise to call her twice in one week. "Not another man who promises and does not deliver!" Amy forcefully told him to get lost. When he left, she fell into despair and cried herself to sleep nightly for a week. "The entire affair lasted 30 days."

"How long do I have to go through this pain of wanting to see him?" We began to focus on the conditions in her life that enabled her to find this handsome, fun-loving, repeatedly unfaithful man the answer to her midlife worries. "My mother says I have always had terrible judgment when it came to men."

Love in a Committed Relationship

Falling in love is a relatively easy topic to understand. Its brief dramatic moments have been the object of much excellent fiction, biography, and discourse. The clarity of love pretty much stops there for me. I find the rest, although much commented on, fascinatingly baffling. Sometimes in retrospect therapists find themselves saying, "Your love was doomed from the beginning!" or pronouncing something like, "Only if two people are at the same developmental level can love flourish!" I am wary of such certainty.

Lasting, ever-deepening love is much admired but rarely studied. Clearly, members of our society have great trouble keeping the quieter affectionate, harmonious, mutually enhancing love of earlier dreams alive. Such "mature" love requires some sort of balance between self and other that eludes many people. I like to think of this joint venture as requiring the ability to put the other ahead of the self at key moments.

Therapists have an opportunity to see the enormous variety of patterns within long-term relationships. We can easily occupy ourselves for a professional lifetime trying to discern and articulate the forces that govern loving relationships. Many of our patients are failing at translating their will to love into behavior that is experienced as caring by the partner. They look to us for assistance, suggestions, explanations—anything—that might reasonably put a stop to their inability to love and be loved by their mate. Clinicians need not be embarrassed at being a lifelong student of love; it is one of the benefits of the work!

Individuals and couples frequently bring their strained love in a committed relationship to psychotherapy. The symptoms that are the initial focus of attention may not be sexual in nature, but sexual constraints are usually lurking. In thinking about the causes of sexual desire disorders— both of the inhibited and the excessive varieties—clinicians should not fail to consider the obvious as the explanation for a couple's problems: they do not love each other. On the other hand, the couple's presence in the professional's office is an invitation to help them consider how this once promising love evolved to the point where they are now considering the relationship relatively loveless.

SUMMARY

Sexual desire is riddled with paradox. It is comprised of three components which often urge us in opposite directions. Sexual desire is a key concept in understanding all of sexuality; it is integral to both sexual identity and function. It is much easier to define sexual desire as the mental force that propels people toward physical intimacies than it is to understand the causes of persistent avoidance of sexual experiences. Many of these problems, now diagnosed as inhibited sexual desire, initially appear to be of obscure etiology. Some yield their mystery to the realization that there is a fundamental lack of respect for the partner, a poor fit of sexual identities, or negative parental transferences to the partner. Still other problems seem to have been brought on by a deepening commitment to a partner, which caused an abandonment of some basic erotic script dominated by lustlike aggressive intensity.

Sexual desire contributes to our understanding of love and love to our understanding of desire. Our concepts of ideal psychological health demand that sexual desire be experienced in the context of affection, which may or may not have been initiated with a passionate beginning. Passionate beginnings may be largely irrelevant to what happens in the future when the couple has to deal with their continuing personal development and struggles to balance their individual needs with those of the partner. How well the couple deals with ongoing challenges may determine whether sexual desire is maintained or fades away.

REFERENCES

1. Kaplan HS: *Disorders of Sexual Desire*. New York, Brunner/Mazel, 1979.
2. Spector IP, Carey MP: Incidence and prevalence of the sexual dysfunctions: A critical review of the literature. *Archives of Sexual Behavior*, 1990; 19:389–408.
3. Bancroft J: *Human Sexuality and Its Problems*, 2nd ed. Edinburgh, Churchill Livingstone, 1989, pp 201–211, 360–372.
4. Regier DA, Boyd J, Burke JD, et al: One-month prevalence of mental disorders in the United States: Based on five epidemiologic catchment area sites. *Archives of General Psychiatry*, 1988; 45:977–986.
5. Warner P, Bancroft J, et al: A regional service for sexual problems: A 3-year study. *Sexual and Marital Therapy*, 1987; 2:115–126.
6. Pomerantz SM: Neurotransmitter influences on male sexual behavior of rhesus monkeys. Read before the IASR, Barrie, Ontario, August 1991.
7. Foreman MM, Hall JL, Love RL: The role of 5-HT-2 receptor in the regulation of sexual performance of male rats. *Life Sciences*, 1989; 45:1263–1270.
8. Segraves, RT: The effects of psychotropic drugs on human erection and ejaculation. *Archives of General Psychiatry*, 1989; 46:275–284.
9. Sherwin BB, Gelfand MM: The role of androgen in the maintenance of sexual functioning in oophorectomized women. *Psychosomatic Medicine*, 1987; 49:397–409.
10. Friedman, R: *Male Homosexuality: A Modern Psychoanalytic Perspective*. New Haven, Yale University Press, 1989.
11. Weinrich JD: *Sexual Landscapes: Why We Are What We Are, Why We Love Whom We Love*. New York, Charles Scribner's Sons, 1987.
12. Freud, S: On the universal tendency to debasement in the sphere of love (Contributions to

the Psychology of Love II), in Strachey, L (ed): *Standard Edition of the Complete Works of Sigmund Freud Vol XI*. London, Hogarth Press, 1912, pp 179–190.

13. Viederman M: The nature of passionate love, in Gaylin W, Person E (eds): *Passionate Attachments: Thinking about Love*. New York, The Free Press, 1988, pp 1–14.

14. Person ES: *Dreams of Love and Fateful Encounters: The Power of Romantic Passion*. New York, WW Norton, 1988.

CHAPTER 6

Preparing to Conduct Therapy

Clinical work is far more complicated than our theories. Our interventions are far less immediately helpful than we like to admit.

AN EXAMPLE OF A ONE-HOUR EVALUATION IN THE IMPOTENCE CLINIC

The Wife's Story as It Was Revealed

Because the urologist was seeing the patient when I was available, I interviewed the wife for the first half hour. From her initial sentences, this middle-aged social service worker was cleaning up her language: "Dan says he gets as much pleasure from having sex as he does from taking . . . moving his bowels." Although they now had intercourse from twice a week to twice a month, he often complained of indifference and limited penile sensations with an occasional loss of erections. She said she had misinterpreted Dan's wanting to hold her in the beginning of their relationship—she was pleased that he was not like other men in that he did not pressure her for intercourse. After they lived together and his sexual avoidance persisted, he suggested that dressing sexier at home would help. After she complied, he lashed out at her for pressuring him to have sex. "Sometimes he is impossible. I could have sex daily, that is not the problem. He keeps talking about how it used to be; he wants to be a 20-year-old again!"

They have been a couple for 6 years, married for 2; recently they ended a 6-month separation. During their premarital days, he was unfaithful at least twice, but she had no further details. "During our separation I realized he was the first man I really loved. But if he doesn't want to be married, it is okay, I'll survive. I can take care of myself." She left because of Dan's mood swings and poor communication. "We would be having a nice time together then suddenly he starts calling me "bitch" and blaming me: "You don't turn me on." "You hate my kids." "You think you are better than me." When she finally left, he was ignoring her, paying no regard to her feelings or presence.

To my surprise, she shifted in her chair and said that she better "cut out the bullshit" and tell me what was going on: "Dan's marriage broke up when he was discovered to be molesting his daughter. I am an incest survivor. I work with survivors all day long. When he is with his daughter, things are not kosher. He looks at her wrong. She dresses real sexy around him. When she got married recently, he really bent over backwards to be nice to her. She and I have recently had some good talks about incest. I told her she should have therapy. I see all the patterns in her."

I encouraged her to tell me what she thought was the underlying problem. "I think Dan can't get excited because he is trying not to get excited about her." She did not know how long the incest lasted, what it consisted of, or how it was discovered. To emphasize how little he communicates, she described the mystery he created about himself by repeatedly saying, "There is something you need to know about me," without telling her. Finally, he said, "There was incest," but would not discuss it.

A note on his medical report indicated a past low testosterone level. She told me that Dan refused to take the treatment the doctor prescribed for it.

She decided to return to him 3 months ago, after he began seeing a counselor and, without her prodding, apologized to her children for his prior cruelty and false accusations. He seemed to take more responsibility for his behavior. He stopped seeing the therapist shortly after he moved back in with her.

The Husband's Story as It Was Revealed

I then spent another half hour with him, a tall, muscular, handsome, matter-of-fact, oilfield worker. He initially spoke of the period between 18 and 36 years of age when he was horny all the time, had sex one way or another once or twice a day, and responded with erection to the sight of women on the street, in magazines, or videos. Now that he is 43, he feels "like a steer—a castrated bull." "I just don't find my wife sexy. Something is wrong because when we separated I went to Texas to work and never once even tried to have a woman. She didn't believe me."

I commented that people can be quite depressed after a marriage breaks up, especially a second marriage; such feelings rob people of their sexual interest. "Yes, I was bummed out, I felt depressed." After his divorce at age 35, he pursued women all the time. During our conversation, he inched his way to speaking of these partners as pieces of ass, one of whom he used to be with only for 15 minutes for sex. "It was great." When he met his wife-to-be, however, things were different. "I can't explain it, but she wasn't a bimbo. She had qualities, you know. I respected her. I was never too interested in sex with her."

He told me that he had never had any interest in anything kinky. Always heterosexual, he thought that some of that way-out stuff like bondage and rape was really sick. He laughed and said maybe he had a lingerie fetish, but no more than other men. He still felt a strong desire for sex and was horny about twice a week, but not like the old days and not for his wife. Children did not interest him as sexual partners.

I told him that his wife told me of her incest with her father and his with his daughter. His eyes opened wider for a moment. Calmly, he told me that it was not what it seemed. He only fondled his daughter's breasts and never had intercourse. His first wife, however, had "forever" been unfaithful to him and even got pregnant by another man. He, too, had been unfaithful. "After a while, I basically ignored her." When the incest was discovered, she found a way to get out of the marriage by appearing to be lily-white. "I went to jail for a month, to counseling for 2 months, and then had trouble obtaining good jobs. This thing still shows up in my life. I have a good relationship with my daughter." He denied that the memory of their sexual interactions was ever on his mind or that he was suppressing his desire in order to be excited by his daughter.

The Brief Meeting with the Couple

The aim of this brief evaluation was to make a tentative diagnosis and prescribe a pathway of therapy. I told the couple that I thought his sexual complaints were explained by his sexual desire problem: his lifelong inability to bring his sexual self to any woman for whom he felt respect and affection. I reassured him that all the physical parameters of his examination were normal, including his testosterone, and recommended individual psychotherapy in their distant rural community. I offered to discuss his situation with a therapist of his choosing.

A brief discussion ensued about his previous therapist's being a coworker of his wife. I agreed that he should not have therapy with any friend of his wife. Her face expressed her skepticism that her minor acquaintance with his counselor explained his leaving therapy.

BACK TO THE BEGINNING—WHY NOW?

People seek out a clinician for symptoms that they consider a problem. Their request for help can be more incisively understood by asking the questions, "Why now?" "What made you decide to come now for help?" Many patients may be uncertain about answering. They may not have clearly considered the question before, they may be frightened by the answer, or they may sense that the answer puts them in an unfavorable light. Sexual problems are often brought to the clinician when one person no longer seems to be able to participate emotionally in the relationship. The "Why now?" answer is that the existence of the relationship is threatened. When the clinician can help a person articulate the major complaints and "Why now?" the therapist is on track and the patient knows it.

Dan's symptoms had been present for 6 years. His wife's preparedness to permanently leave him produced his visit. It remains to be seen whether his efforts to attain assistance are sincere or another ploy to stall and placate his wife.

BEYOND THE DIAGNOSIS

The therapist's initial listening is geared to recognizing diagnostic categories in the patient's complaints. I thought Dan's multiply impaired sexual function was parsimoniously understood by his need to avoid sexual behavior. His inhibited sexual desire appeared to me to correspond to the fourth item in this list of causes of inhibited sexual desire:

1. Lack of respect for the partner
2. Unmet gender, orientation, or intention needs
3. Negative transference
4. Inability to love and have sex with the same person
5. Inability to love the partner

Diagnosis is important, of course, but it has limitations. This list of "causes" of inhibited sexual desire suggests that there is no overlap between these categories; this could not be correct. Diagnoses and differential diagnoses are conventions used by professionals so that their therapies point in a helpful direction. Once therapy begins in earnest, the diagnosis or the understanding of its meaning often changes. There is always more to a person's sexual and emotional life than can be captured by any diagnosis—sexual or psychiatric.

A longer, more systematized psychiatric evaluation of Dan might have yielded a further description such as:

- Axis I—Inhibited Sexual Desire
- Axis II—Sociopathic Personality
- Axis III—Herniated Lumbar 4–5 Disc
- Axis IV—Intense Stress of Marital and Intrafamilial Discord
- Axis V—Highest Level of Adaptive Functioning—60

Beyond formal sexual or psychiatric diagnostic processes, the therapist has to continually return to two questions: "What is the problem here?" and "What can I do about it?" These are *big* questions—that is, they should not be expected to be glibly answered. Rather, the therapist should expect to reconsider these questions periodically throughout the relationship to the patient.

WHAT CONSTITUTES A SEXUAL PROBLEM?

On the surface, this is a needless question because the answer is that sexual symptoms constitute the sexual problem. When people have disruptions of their sexual psychophysiology, they, by definition, have sexual problems. The clinician skillfully elicits the complaints, decides whether they involve gender identity struggles, paraphilic interests, or dysfunctional responses, and designates a formal nosologic category. The formula is simple: the symptoms = the problem. After a little clinical experience, this DSM-III-R-oriented task is easily mastered.

When the goal of diagnosis is treatment planning, however, the question of what constitutes a sexual problem is far from simple. Clinicians think about sexual symptoms differently depending on their cause. In our early evaluation hours with patients, we follow two guiding principles: (1) symptoms signify underlying pathophysiology or disease; (2) whenever possible, treatment should be directed at the cause not the symptoms. As we sift through the possibilities that organic, personal, interpersonal, and cultural factors may be contributing to a person's symptoms, we are no longer equating symptoms with problems.

The therapeutic challenges to mental health clinicians posed by sexual symptoms vary dramatically according to the cause of the symptom and according to nonsexual aspects of the patient. In the next section, I want to address how clinicians' perceptions of cause influence whether sexual symptoms are dignified as sexual problems. In the following section, I want to deal with how nonsexual factors determine treatability.

SHOULD CAUSE DEFINE PROBLEMS?

Organically Induced Sexual Symptoms

Sexual symptoms may be caused by nonsexual organic disease processes. Hormonal deficiencies, spinal cord injuries, medication effects, or congestive heart failure, for example, can readily generate sexual symptoms. The consequences of organically induced sexual symptoms may be psychosocially profound—for example, ovarian failure in a young woman can cause her psychological and relationship problems. These consequences follow from the organic pathophysiology.

Dyspareunia, or pain during intercourse, a symptom that precludes relaxed arousal during intercourse, is sometimes due to an organic illness called *endometriosis*. The consequences of persistent dyspareunia can render a couple asexual, create a pattern of guilt and anger in both partners, and eventually play in important role in the dissolution of their relationship. The woman's pain may be relieved by surgically removing the aberrant patch of endometrial tissue or administering a hormone that suppresses the growth of this tissue. Because dyspareunia caused by endometriosis is an organic problem, it is usually cared for by gynecologists without referral to mental health professionals, despite its frequent psychosexual consequences. To the patient, pain is a serious and threatening problem—a sexual problem; to the gynecologist, dyspareunia is the symptom, endometriosis is the problem. This is exactly how the medical model operates. Disease produces symptoms. Treatment is directed at the underlying illness.

Psychosocially Induced Sexual Symptoms

These symptoms are viewed differently; they are now felt to be relatively discrete, unidimensional difficulties experienced in the sphere of sexual function alone. Their existence does not imply the presence of other problematic spheres of mental functioning. For example, an anorgasmic woman is not necessarily unfriendly, unloving, an alcoholic, nervous in public places, or paranoid; she just cannot attain orgasm. When a clinician judges the anorgasmia to be due to a combination of educational deficits, guilt over personal pleasures, and limiting concepts of women's roles, the symptom is likely to be thought of as a genuine sexual dysfunction. The perception of a genuine sexual dysfunction is related to the inability to quickly identify a convincing psychosocial cause.

Our culture currently thinks that there are specific treatments for sexual dysfunctions. Beginning therapists, however, need to quickly understand that effective treatment cannot be reduced to a universally applied sequence of steps. Treatment contains many elements—such as exploration of developmental meanings of the problem, education, encouragement, practicing sexual exercises, and identification with the therapist. The few techniques that we possess are applied in a distinctive human–human interaction which creates a uniqueness of content, sequence, and style.

The goal of therapy for psychosexual dysfunctions is generally similar from one patient to the next: enable or restore ordinary physiological functioning. For lifelong anorgasmic women, for example, therapy is aimed at helping them to realize their biological capacity to experience intense arousal for their own sake. Anorgasmia may be treated in individual or in group therapy, and is usually the province of mental health professionals who feel particularly educated about sexuality. In prior decades, anorgasmia and other orgasmic problems were considered symptoms of a disease called *neurosis*, which was perceived to have other manifestations as well. Fashions in diagnosis and preferred explanations of cause have changed.

Sexual Symptoms Caused by Childhood Sexual Experience

If a person's symptom—for instance, vaginismus or erectile unreliability with partners—is recognized to be a consequence of coerced childhood sexual victimization, clinicians think about the patient's sexual deficits differently. The dysfunctions are thought of as symptoms of a posttraumatic stress disorder, a dissociative disorder, a paraphilia, or a negative transference problem. These dysfunctions are thought of as deeper, more serious problems than genuine sexual dysfunctions and are perceived to be associated with other emotional problems. The therapist's attention is drawn more toward dealing with the traumatic childhood experiences and the affects, meanings, and coping strategies employed by the victim over time rather than by specific techniques for overcoming the symptom. The consequences of childhood sexual abuse are cared for by various mental health professionals with and without a special educational background in sexuality or victimology.

Two objections to these professional attitudes can be raised: the sexual deficits of people with a more "benign" pathogenesis are as dysfunctional as those who were sexually victimized as children; in pursuing the childhood trauma, the mental health professional often ignores the sexual symptoms.

Sexual Symptoms Caused by Relationship Problems

Many desire, arousal, and orgasm problems are best explained by the nonsexual interactions of two people, each of whom has been, and is capable of, adequate sexual function. Many therapists do not even consider these to be sexual problems. The sexual deficits are assumed to by the symptoms of the couple's interpersonal problem. A variety of mental health professionals offer marital therapy. After the initial evaluation, sexual symptoms may never be mentioned. The error that is frequently made with distressed couples is to assume that their sexual life has deteriorated from a normal to its dysfunctional sexual level as a result of their interpersonal conflict. The presumption misses the large number of distressed couples who under the best of times were limited by sexual dysfunction.

Character-Disorder-Driven Sexual Symptoms

Some sexual symptom clusters appear to be a product of some other basic pattern in a person. Generally, clinicians do not do well in articulating exactly what this is, but we think they relate to deficits in integrity, intelligence, self-esteem, maturity, or character. For instance, Dan might be thought of as possessing a limited capacity to feel responsible for the interpersonal chaos he helps to create. In character-disorder-driven sexual dysfunctions, the sexual symptoms are usually perceived to be related to other aspects of mental functioning.

Dan's sexual symptoms were quickly appraised by me as part of an array of problems—marital discord, irresponsibility, infidelity, incest, lying, and sadistic treatment of family members. I leaned toward thinking about him as closely resembling the mode of a sociopathic character disorder, even though I did not ascertain this Axis II diagnosis in a deliberate fashion.

Causal explanations about a person's character disorder involve something pervasive yet intangible in the personality. A person whose anxiety about rejection prevents arousal with a partner is often considered to have a sexual problem that is due to low self-esteem. The low self-esteem is assumed to have many manifestations in the person's thinking and behavior. Sexual dysfunction is the focus only because of the patient's presentation. Characterologically driven sexual problems are the province of psychotherapists. These sexual problems are also easily lost in the attempt to help these persons with their more basic problems.

There is no compelling reason to think that only the character-disordered have psychogenic dysfunctions caused by their basic personality organization. Even those of us who are not perceived by diagnosticians as having an Axis II diagnosis have sexual symptoms whose roots extend into our character organization. Character organization mediates the development of sexual symptoms through recurrent behavioral traits—character traits—and through internal images of other people.

Character is manifested by recurrent, reasonably dependable behavioral traits that accompany us through various developmental phases of life. Here is a far-from-complete list of behavioral traits that play a role in the origin of some people's sexual symptoms: passivity, entitlement, fearfulness of emotional intensity, self-centeredness, selflessness, fearfulness of disapproval, controlling, competitiveness. When clinicians describe a sexually dysfunctional person with such words, there is a good chance that these traits play a role in the symptom's origin or maintenance.

Much of our psychology, of course, is dependent on unseen but deducible aspects of ourselves. When the unseen aspects of personality are discussed, mental health professionals are using theoretical notions. These ideas have great currency in our field, produce ideology and its controversies, and help clinicians to create an identity. Here is a bare-bones notion that clinicians often use to explain the relationship between character and symptoms: We behave toward our significant others in terms of our internalized images of them. The inability to react to each person based on their actual behavior—that is, our tendency to be too trusting, frightened, aggressive, or cynical—can be understood by what we have originally incorporated into our psyches about close relationships with family members. Object relations theory emphasizes that sexual symptoms are more a reflection of internalized images of the relationship between self and others than of other factors. One of the favorite explanations of object relations theorists is *splitting*, the defense mechanism that too quickly and too often separates people into good and bad parts, making it difficult to act as though the person is composed of both strengths and weaknesses. Some people view their spouses as "bad objects" as soon as the first major frustration occurs. This private new view of the spouse becomes the basis for global or sexual rejection, which, in turn, leads to a variety of sexual symptoms. The disturbances of internalized object relations are more easily perceived among the character-disordered than among the characterologically normal people with sexual dysfunction, but are not unique to them.

This fifth category of problems also follows a medical model—the sexual dysfunctions are symptoms and the organization of character is the underlying disorder. In fact, four of the five categories view the dysfunctions as symptoms of some basic underlying defect—such as biology, interpersonal relationships, childhood trauma, and internal object relationships. Only the "genuine" sexual dysfunctions have yet to attract a more substantial causal explanation. As we shall continue to see, genuine sexual dysfunction is an illusion. All psychogenic sexual dysfunction is genuine.

Clinical resolution of the tensions between the simple and the causal view of sexual symptoms is possible. To the patient, each of these five categories of sexual symptoms are sexual problems. The equation, symptoms = problems, cannot be forgotten by clinicians just because we need also to be preoccupied with causes. Our role is to help people do better with what they consider a problem. To a large extent, we are judged by our patients by the degree to which we are concerned with their symptoms. If we have a better view of the symptom, one that convincingly explains it, we should offer our perspective to the patient for consideration. It is, of course, ideal, if our explanation sets the stage for curing the problem. The everpresent danger from our preoccupation with cause, however, is redefining the problem in a way that ignores the patient's distress.

THE TREATABILITY OF PEOPLE WITH SEXUAL SYMPTOMS

Is the Patient Treatable?

Medical doctors tend to refer their patients for psychotherapeutic help when psychogenic sexual dysfunctions are present. They rarely send their patients who have conspicuous organically caused dysfunctions. There are several ironies here: just because a problem is psychogenic does not mean that it is treatable with psychotherapy; just because a dysfunction has been initiated by an organic factor does not mean that a mental health professional could not be of help. The relationship between causality and treatability should be better understood by mental health professionals than it is by nonpsychiatric physicians.

Albert

A rational, masculine, heterosexual lawyer, Albert knows it is his fault that his marriage has been unconsummated for 12 years. He cannot bring himself to initiate lovemaking but has no idea why, except that he is a procrastinator. Albert is polite, friendly, affectless, and unable to recall his childhood. He is boring as many compulsive people are for therapists; I have to work to ask him questions, and he has difficulty elaborating on anything. His ideal is constant emotional stability—he wants to be a straight line, no wavering with intensity of any kind. Even his weekly masturbation is undertaken to prevent sexual feelings rather than to respond to them.

Albert loves his wife, finds her very attractive, far more than his "nerdy" self should physically deserve, he adds. He is afraid he will someday lose her, but dread has not been enough to change his behavior. He intellectually wants to have sex but something stops him. When his wife initiates lovemaking, he does better but always loses his erection sometime during their foreplay. "I guess I wouldn't mind if we didn't have sex; I am a take-it-or-leave-it person, although I am very embarrassed about it. Anyway, this is definitely not normal!"

Albert wanted to come to therapy every 3 to 4 weeks. "I can't afford more!" I reluctantly agreed to see him twice each month; he was unable to schedule his fourth session because he forgot his calendar and was not heard from again for 4 months. He then began weekly sessions.

After 4 years of 2 to 4 times-a-month therapy with Albert, alone and sometimes with his wife, the relationship is still not consummated, although Albert is more aware of his affects, sexual feelings, and the sources of his inhibition. He now touches his wife intimately occasionally.

Patient Factors

Albert had trouble using his sessions. He waited for me to bring up topics and to explain answers to his rare questions. He offered little from the events between sessions. He preferred to talk about legal problems or to watch the building being constructed outside of my window. I spent much of my time teaching him to label his muted affects and helping him not to change the subject when they arose. He remembered almost nothing about his family experiences and could only provide a minimal sketch of his parents—a normal, devoted, hard-working, father and an unpredictable mother who sometimes seemed off the wall. "I don't know" was his most common answer. Albert's mind often went blank during our sessions. I had to constantly remind myself that he was not processing during our silences; he was only waiting for me to bring up the next subject. He often did not think about our conversations between sessions. Eventually, I asked to have his wife come with him so that I could learn about his family. That proved helpful for me—and the sessions were lively.

Michelle possessed an intense reactivity to her mother-in-law. Albert's retreat from emotions seemed to make sense when Michelle gave numerous examples of his mother's rages, ranting, and intrusiveness into each of her children's lives. Albert's annoyance when his nightly retreat into reading was disturbed sounded like the continuation of his coping with his mother (who was recently diagnosed as manic-depressive, although inadequately treated). I thought Albert suffered from a negative transference from his mother to Michelle.

Clinicians quickly learn two lessons once they begin with therapy. The forces that motivate a person for a consultation are not necessarily the same that enable the patient to use therapy well. And sexual dysfunction is not always simple to overcome.

Dan, a man with a character disorder, and Albert, a man with an obsessive-compulsive personality style, both have the same dysfunction—inhibited sexual desire. It is neither the symptoms nor the diagnosis that can make effective therapy possible or unworkable. Patients' motives, intellectual capacities, comfort with their inner lives, style of being in the world, defenses, and partners also affect treatability. When a person possesses a profile of factors that suggest a difficult therapy, the treatment should be undertaken with an awareness that the treatment will not be easy, simply educational, or readily accomplished in a fixed number of sessions. Such realism prevents the patient from being misled about obtaining a "quick fix" and buffers the therapist from feeling incompetent when the patient continues to be dysfunctional after many months.

Clinicians often say that the patient has to be motivated to work in therapy. This means that the patient has to (1) have a belief in the therapy's potential for helping; (2) have a modest capacity to be an intimate speaker; (3) have courage to face unpleasant moments; (4) have patience to stay until better or there is no current possibility of improvement; (5) believe there is a personal role in the genesis of the problem; (6) possess the inner sense that life would be significantly better if the symptoms could be removed; (7) have the financial means to pay for therapy; and (8) (if married) have a spouse who is supportive of the therapy and will privately view improvement as a personal benefit.

Many psychotherapies, in private and institutional settings alike, stop before they have a chance to develop. Even though the therapist has been skillful, early dropout occurs because of some combinations of patient factors.

Therapist Factors That Facilitate Therapy

The therapist has to possess some of the same factors that are required of the patient. Therapists have to have (1) a belief in the therapy's capacity to help; (2) intimacy listening skills; (3) courage to pay attention to what is happening within their mental privacy and to speak honestly to the patient; (4) patience to keep at the work of therapy; (5) an intuitive grasp of the relationship between the past and the present; and (6) a sense of the therapeutic process.

Although progress and even "cure" are possible for many people who have sexual problems, many others do not improve during their therapies. Therapy can be useful, nonetheless, in helping them to recognize what prevents them from losing their symptoms. Clinicians need to walk a fine line between vigilant work—that is, conceptualizing the problem and processing relevant affects—and the recognition that too much has transpired in the person's life to simply get better.

Barbara

Barbara's 35th birthday present to herself was a consultation about her sexual life. She and her very kind husband had had almost no sexual interaction since their last child was born a decade ago. Barbara had sexual drive, motive, and wish. She thought she could get aroused, but it had been a long time. She had never had an orgasm by any means. A couples therapy ensued. Her husband went through the motions of lovemaking to please her but had no interest in it for mysterious reasons (our concepts about the causes of sexual desire disorders were not as advanced then). After 6 months, we abandoned our efforts with a sense of hopelessness about their capacity to be sexual as a couple.

Several months later, Barbara returned to discuss her anorgasmia. She began working hard at overcoming her inhibitions and learned how to attain orgasm with masturbation. She established a relationship with another man but was anorgasmic. During her psychotherapy, she continued to discuss her self-induced restraints during physical intimacies. Three months into a new relationship with a divorced man, Barbara began to regularly attain orgasms during genital touching and intercourse. Barbara's asexual marriage has persisted for almost two decades since the failure of couples therapy. She and her lover periodically meet, make love, and enjoy her easy orgasmic attainment.

A Brief Intervention for an Organically Impaired Man

Benjamin, a 73-year-old retired businessman, had been treated for 8 months with a gonadotropin-blocking agent since his mastectomy for cancer. The medical goal was to keep his testosterone level at a minimal level and minimize the risk of metastasis. Benjamin was informed that he must stay on Tomaxafin for the rest of his life. He had enjoyed an excellent sexual life for his 48 years of marriage. Even now that he lost his potency and much of his usually vigorous drive, he had the wish to have a better sexual life. He decreased the frequency of sexual initiations for fear he was going to be impotent. He felt he could not discuss the matter with his wife because he was too humiliated by his lost abilities. She, generally orgasmic with intercourse, mouth, or hand stimulation, had stopped any initiation. He requested a referral about his sexual life from his oncologist.

Benjamin had a three-visit "cure," despite a testosterone reading of 174 ng/dL. I expressed doubt that he was entirely unable to have intercourse despite the fact that he had no erections of any lasting duration since the Tomaxafin. I told him that testosterone was more important for fantasy formation than erection maintenance. I emphasized that the major current problems were his avoidance of sexual experience for fear of impotence and his sexual deprivation of his wife without so much as an explanation. I sent him home with instructions to make love without trying to have intercourse three times over the following month. At his next visit, he reported that they had made love twice. Each time, his wife had an orgasm and he had an elongated but soft erection. He had begun lovemaking each time without discussion. He reported that on one occasion, he had a stand-up morning erection, but following my advice, he did not attempt to use it for intercourse. I repeated my instructions—no intercourse until he had made love three more times, but this time he had to discuss his visit to me with his wife. Eight weeks later, he was a much happier man. His wife was delighted to have returned to lovemaking. She told him how much she had missed their closeness and how afraid she was of making his ordeal with cancer worse. They had made love six times—the fourth and last time intercourse had occurred. "I'm not thirty any more; it was good enough!"

By dint of their ambition to have a better sexual life, Barbara and Benjamin were able to reverse conditions that render most people asexual. They stand as examples of patient factors beyond diagnosis and cause that account for treatability.

SUMMARY

Although patients and professionals alike may think of a clinician who deals directly with sexual problems as a "sex doctor," it is difficult to ignore the embedding of sexual symptoms in other biological, social, and psychological phenomena. Sex doctors have to be as competent as general mental health professionals and have an appreciation of the limitations of fashionable concepts about sexual problems. In their own eyes, clinicians quickly cease being sex doctors and become diagnosticians, individual psychotherapists, marital psychotherapists, and counselors. The goal remains to try to understand the source of sexual symptoms and what can be done to ameliorate them. This requires the mental health clinician to play many roles, beginning with thoughtful diagnosis, moving to understanding the requirements for therapy-induced changes, and forever remaining a student of the complexity of sexuality. Sex doctors have a lifetime of professional opportunity to think about the many factors that interfere with the will to love and be loved. All psychotherapists can be sex, relationship, and love doctors if they will open their eyes and stop dismissing sexual dysfunction as a mere symptom.

CHAPTER 7

The Sexual Equilibrium

The sexual equilibrium is the most misunderstood influence on sexual life. Within it, with lightning speed, the partners' regard for each other often seals their fate.

THE ESSENCE IS BALANCE

Besides being influenced by a host of nonsexual factors—affective, cognitive, interpersonal, social, biological, and developmental—sexual life also exists in an arena all by itself. It has a life of its own. This life takes place in a psychological realm where additional interactions shape sexual experience. In previous publications, I have labeled the arena the *sexual equilibrium* because balance between the partners is its essence.[1]

The balance, which is unseen but felt, either creates sexual comfort or discomfort. When the equilibrium routinely generates comfort for both partners, the couple feels enhanced, enjoys their intimate physical behaviors, and returns to them frequently. When the equilibrium consistently induces disappointment, they feel diminished and return to sexual opportunity less often.

WHAT IS BALANCED?

Two major forces are balanced in the sexual equilibrium: the component characteristics of each partner and the regard each person has for the partner's component characteristics.

The Interplay of Components

The three components of each partner's sexual identity have a dramatic interplay in the beginning of a couple's relationship. Because sexual identity plays a role in partner choice and sexual activity, some couples with major incompatibilities of identity do not last as a couple because one of them does not fit with the other—they discover their imbalance early in their couplehood. This problem can, of course, be discussed, but often is not. A homoerotic previously homosexual woman, for example, may not choose to tell a man why she does not want to make love or why love-making is not pleasing to her. She just may let the relationship die a mysterious-to-the-man death. Clinicians often hear about partners who lack sexual desire; it is usually up to them to figure out that the explanation is an imbalance of gender identities, orientation, or intention.

Sexual desire discrepancies are often symptoms of imbalances or in-compatibilities of the six sexual components. These may involve the sexual identity or sexual function components. When a man has trouble relaxing, maintaining an erection, or becoming sensuous, his partner may quickly become unable to be aroused with him and may lose motivation to make love. When one partner initiates lovemaking four times a week and the partner responds receptively only weekly, their imbalanced desire shapes their chronic frustration on both of their parts.

Of course, sexual function components can be highly compatible. The woman who is easily orgasmic sexually can get along well with a host of partners, whether they are readily orgasmic or not. When two people have similar drive frequencies, sexual accommodation does not become a major issue between them. There is a broad range of compatibilities of sexual components among couples. To the extent that a couple's identity and function components are highly incompatible, their sexual equilibrium will be more difficult to maintain over time.

The interaction of sexual component characteristics is not something that occurs a few times early in the life of a couple and is forever fixed at the balance that is attained. The interplay is constantly occurring because the component characteristics evolve over time. Our desire, arousal, and orgasmic capacities fluctuate a great deal more than our identity charac-teristics, but all six have their own rhythms of fluctuation. The sexual equilibrium is a *dynamic* balance of forces.

Regard

Regard is an attitude. It may be displayed verbally or behaviorally. Either way it reflects personal judgment about whether something is ac-ceptable. Regard is the second key factor that is balanced within the sexual equilibrium. Once personal judgments produce regard, these crucial steps take place in each partner: (1) a person perceives how the partner regards what one is or does sexually; (2) the perception of regard either increases personal abandon or increases inhibition; (3) if abandonment to sensuality occurs, positive attitudes toward the self and the partner are stabilized; and

(4) if the growth of self-consciousness occurs, negative attitudes toward the self and the partner evolve.

The existence of the sexual equilibrium is easy to miss. Even when it is pointed out, it may be initially difficult to grasp. The interplay of sexual component characteristics and how they are regarded are subtle and rapid. They also occur simultaneously in each partner. When what actually transpires in this sexual arena is first acknowledged, some clinicians dismiss it as too superficial an explanation for our sexual fates. They prefer explanations that feel more profound and powerful. We must be careful here. Sexuality is constantly being explained away by nonsexual issues. I am not arguing that the sexual equilibrium explains everything about our sexual fate. It does seem to explain some phenomena, however.

> Attractive Maggie has one of the most hateful attitudes toward a husband I have ever witnessed. When alone together, or in front of the children, or with her best women friends, Maggie's disgust for Eric's weakness, lying, and failure to earn as much as other husbands, and his inability to stand up to his father, knows no limits of expression. In conjoint therapy, she speaks of him in the same I-can't-stand-to-even-look-at-you manner. She readily lapses into a litany of his failures as a human being.
>
> "But, I can say one good thing about Eric, he is good in bed!" Their frequent mutual orgasmic sexual activity is impervious to her attacks and his sense that he is going to lose his mind, if she does not stop. Easily aroused, sex-loving Maggie is a recovered agoraphobic with persistent driving and work phobias. Eric is a passive-aggressive, indecisive man with poor judgment who contemplates suicide on occasion. When their marital and intrapsychic woes reached a fever pitch—Eric's business reversals and Maggie's panic about losing her beauty and her terror of having no role in life when her baby left for college— their frequent satisfying sexual life continued without missing a beat. Laughing in the midst of their gloom, each shrugs and says, "It is the one thing we have always had going for us."

The sexual equilibria that clinicians usually hear about are problematic, but Maggie and Eric are an illuminating exception. Once clinicians acknowledge that sexual life is important unto itself and understand how the components and the regard for them interact, they begin hearing patients talking about their dilemmas concerning their partner's sexual traits. "If I speak about my reactions, I may hurt my partner deeply. If I do not speak, I have to endure and hope for the best, but I know that I cannot tolerate this."

PROBLEMATIC SEXUAL TRAITS

Each partner brings many sexual traits to the bedroom. Clinicians are generally only aware of those that their patients' repeatedly regard negatively. These range widely over many matters: interest in behaving sexually; ease of arousal; ability to have orgasm; talking or not talking during lovemaking; preference for activity or passivity; preference for an intercourse style; desire for mouth–genital stimulation; insistence on cleanliness; clumsiness of vulvar stimulation; and postorgasm sleepiness.

THE SEQUENCE OF REGARD

Step 1: Regard of a Particular Trait

Although clinicians most often hear about the negatively viewed traits, regard ranges widely from enthusiastic pleasure ("I love how excited you get when I caress your breasts!) to comfortable acceptance without comment ("Why should I say anything? Its fine; I have no complaints.") to disappointment without comment ("I wish you would stop lying there waiting for me and get more active!") to harsh criticism ("I hate how you touch me. You are really terrible at this!"). Positive regard has a great deal to do with a good sexual life. Negative regard, whether spoken or not, propels sexual life toward deterioration. The private subjectivity of a sexual partner can contain negative regard without the partner knowing it. However, I suspect that constant, intensely negative regard is much more difficult to hide even from an insensitive partner.

Step 2: Sensual Abandon versus Inhibition

Partner acceptance of what is brought to the bedroom allows the person to relax, to lose self-consciousness, to focus on giving and receiving pleasurable sensations, and gradually to try new sexual behaviors. This allows sex to be an adventure for both partners and sometimes results in ecstatic experiences. It explains why the sexual lives of many couples improve with time.

Partner criticism, especially that which is harshly presented or communicated sharply without discussion, can dramatically limit a person's participation in future sexual activities. When it occurs, a dramatic increase in self-consciousness immediately results which can cripple the potential for personal and partner pleasure.

Step 3: New Attitude to the Self and the Partner

Sexual competence with a partner is highly valued by both sexes. We want to be seen as capable, knowledgeable, and pleasing in our sexual behaviors. The final steps in this three-part sequence are the impact on our gender identity and on our attitude toward our partner. Women feel more feminine if their sexual life works well; men feel more secure in their masculinity when their partner positively regards what transpires. Positive regard from the partner also helps to create the sense that we are loved. Even without the sense that we are loved, positive regard induces a limited but vital happiness.

When the regard is consistently negative, it has the opposite effects. Women privately feel less feminine ("He is never satisfied with me in bed.") and often less attractive ("I'm too fat."). Men feel as though their masculinity is flawed ("I have never been much good at this sex stuff."). Both partners may have to work harder at feeling loved when sexual interactions are negatively regarded. I have never talked to a person who was happy about a dysfunctional sexual life.

Negative regard produces an attack on the self and can also create harsh attitudes toward the partner. It is a simple mental matter, well within the defensive repertoire of most people, to take the perception of personal sexual inadequacy and displace it onto the partner. The result can be increasing resentment toward the partner, which just makes lovemaking more difficult to respond to or initiate.

THE SIGNIFICANCE OF THE SEXUAL EQUILIBRIUM

The sexual equilibrium is useful to clinicians for explaining how a person with a consistent set of sexual characteristics—for instance, rapid ejaculation or slowness to be aroused—can become dysfunctional with one partner and have a happy full sexual life with another. This is a major issue for many people who have participated in unsatisfactory sexual relationships and who are contemplating divorce. Will it be any better with another person? Well, in stark contrast to what some mental health professionals used to promulgate,[2] it certainly can be! The impact of the partner's attitudes toward their sexual style or on their capacity to be relaxed is what enables sex for some couples to be unsatisfying or wonderful. Knowledge of the three-step sequence of the sexual equilibrium provides a road map of the trail followed by couples whose sexual life has ceased entirely. The road traveled to this sad point is often a mystery to patients.

The Sexual Equilibrium and Individual Psychology

In using the concept of the sexual equilibrium, there is no escaping individual psychology. The sexual traits that a person brings to the bedroom sometimes are themselves a product of intrapsychic pain and conflict. For instance, a sexually abused girl may grow up to have limited motivation for any sexual behavior, whereas a sexually abused boy may grow up to have an insignificant desire for his wife relative to his desire for 8-year-old boys.

The regard that a person has for a partner's sexual traits is highly influenced by the hidden meanings that the sexual traits have for each person. For some partners, rapid ejaculation within the vagina means, "I am once again disappointed by life. When will I start getting what I want!" For others, it means, "I find it very exciting that he finds me very exciting." For some men, a woman's pattern of orgasm that is achieved only by clitoral stimulation means, "My penis is too small. Here is yet another example of my inadequate self." For other men, the same pattern provokes only, "I love it when she attains orgasm." In seeking out these meanings and finding longstanding, more profound conflictual themes to explain the impediments to sexual pleasure, clinicians should be wary about losing sight of the rapid, simultaneous, three-step sequence that these meanings subvert.

THE TYPICAL DRAMA AMONG YOUNG COUPLES

I consider rapid ejaculation in the vagina to be a characteristic of the majority of men beginning their experiences with intercourse. Men experience their sudden explosive arousal during intercourse as something that they cannot control. It just happens. Although ejaculation can occur outside the vagina in response to genital touching, the uncontrollable ejaculation drama is typically located in the vagina. Most men get used to the excitement of other forms of genital intimacies faster than they lose their intense arousal during intercourse. The vagina is some special place! Men give themselves some time to get used to intercourse. They intuitively know that this intimacy is both a rite of passage and a badge of masculine competence. While they are patiently waiting for ejaculatory control within the vagina to develop, however, they have impatient, nagging doubts. "How long should it take? We have had intercourse 10 times during the past 2 months!" No sexologist knows for certain how long it should take, but heterosexual men are quick to point out that speed of ejaculation in the vagina depends on age, duration since last orgasm, the degree of arousal prior to entry into the vagina, newness of the partner, and nervousness about having intercourse.

There are three compelling reasons to last longer in the vagina. Men feel an obligation to provide their partner with an opportunity to enjoy the sensations of intercourse; they want to bring the woman to orgasm from thrusting motivations; they want to be as good as other men at this activity. Therapists are not sought out for assistance by men who do not care about their partners' enjoyment, who view intercourse as the male's prize for seduction, or who have intercourse only with prostitutes. Homosexual men almost never ask for help for premature ejaculation. It is the lack of the woman's pleasure, the sense of hopelessly failing to provide a partner with what she needs and deserves, and the fear of being abandoned by the partner that bring coupled men in for help.

Single men contemplating being with a new partner, of course, are concerned with this matter as well. It is they who have anxious anticipation about disgracing themselves and being rejected by their new partner because of their "incompetence" as a sex partner. Here is a clinical case that I have experienced.

> A 22-year-old landscape/snow-plowing assistant was brought in by his girlfriend because of premature ejaculation. Recently, he was unable to thrust more than 2 minutes no matter what position or trick he used—including masturbation to orgasm before they went out together. When they began their sexual relationship 12 months earlier, he lasted longer —10 minutes. His partner was 18, sexually experienced for 2 years with several boyfriends, and absolutely certain about how males should perform. "He is not normal! A woman knows when a man is not normal! He cannot make me come because he squirts off too fast. I don't need to put up with this shit. If you can't fix him, he and I will just forget it." She quickly disagreed with almost everything I had to say. After several interchanges, my hostility must have gotten the best of me. I raised several questions: "Why was orgasm so important that it had to happen every time?" "Why was she so dependent on him for orgasm?" and the cruelest, "What was wrong with 2 minutes of thrusting?" She looked at me like I was a very old person, the wrong person with whom to talk about this.

> I was surprised when they returned. During this last visit, I had myself under better control. They told me a bit about their attachment to each other, which however stormy, was a vast improvement over the chaotic families from which each partner had emerged. He still wants to last at least 10 minutes of vigorous thrusting, as he did when he was into drinking at the beginning of their relationship. He was now in Alcoholics Anonymous. They did not show up for their next appointment.

The Sexual Developmental Task of New Couples

Whatever the dynamics of a couple's newly formed life, the developmental task is the same. They have to establish a way of being sexually intimate together that sufficiently pleases each of them so that negative regard is not palpable. This enables them, of course, to relax and to begin to realize their personal sexual ambitions. For the man, these ambitions usually focus on lasting longer during intercourse and learning how to please the woman before and during intercourse. For the woman, these ambitions usually are to learn how to use her own and his body for her personal pleasure. She may have to instruct him how to please her. If she is too shy, passive, or expectant of him to have all the secrets of how to excite her, she is apt to soon grow weary of his inadequacies and regard him or herself negatively. The young couple is evolving a sexual equilibrium. Each is learning about their sexual responses, their partner's style, and their personal responsibilities to keep the pleasure and intensity going.

New couples do not end up with the same balance of compatibilities and regard. Couples often quietly accept whatever results from their interaction within their sexual equilibrium. Sexual misery should never be defined by the actual sexual limitations within a couple but by their attitudes toward those limitations. One person's cause for misery may not even cause another person any alarm.

The typical problem of the recently sexually active couple, whether married or not, is two-sided: the man ejaculates faster than he or his partner desires and she is unable to have orgasm during their sexual behavior together. Sometimes, this is presented to clinicians as premature ejaculation, sometimes as female anorgasmia, but it actually is a new sexual equilibrium in distress.

Clinical Implications

The idea of looking at the couple as the locus of the problem rather than the apparent symptom bearer was one of the major contributions of Masters and Johnson's pioneering clinical sexologic work during the 1960s.[3] This is a profound idea. If the clinician thinks of the problem as a case of premature ejaculation, one set of responses will likely follow for the male-centered "pathology" (DSM-III-R 302.75). If the clinician thinks of it as a case of anorgasmia, another set of responses will follow for this female-centered "pathology" (DSM-III-R 302.74). If the couple is seen as having a typical problem of new couples, they are apt to be treated as a couple, without the quick application of exercises or a rapid referral for intense psychotherapy.

> Bill, an extremely quiet, soft-spoken, responsible, laboratory technician, a college graduate, son of immigrant uneducated parents, finally found the perfect woman for himself at age 29. He was ecstatic that she loved him. (He conveyed this by saying, "I am very happy" accompanied by a warm, embarrassed, contented smile.) Jane was his first sexual partner. He was devoted to her happiness. Although she was 6 years older and had a good job as a teacher, she was given to "Chicken-Little" perceptions that the sky was falling—"everything is always going wrong." His reasonableness and patience were the clincher in her love for him. She tested him often. Having been in psychotherapy for many years, Jane soon linked this for me to her father's traumatic abandonment of herself and her mother when she was 16. Worry about abandonment had never completely left her. Although she knew this was what was causing her to doubt Bill's stick-to-it-ness, she could not always

counter the worry. Once, she was obsessed for 3 weeks that he was going to be unfaithful like her father because one day after he promised to throw out his *Playboy* magazines, he had not.

Bill initially sought help for premature ejaculation alone. The trouble was that he ejaculated too quickly in Jane's vagina, never outside, and she could not attain orgasm. She had stated emphatically that she could not marry him if she could not have orgasm with him. She was orgasmic with her previous lover, a man 20 years her senior with whom she had broken up a year ago. With him, she had orgasms during intercourse but also plenty of angry, frustration-induced headaches because of his unreliability.

I met Jane on a second visit and saw her and Bill only as a couple. Bill's capacities varied between impotence, premature ejaculation, and 5 minutes of intravaginal movements, seemingly in response to his anxiety about whether he was pleasing her. I was optimistic with them, telling them repeatedly that they had a beautiful loving bond. I thought this was simply a minor coordination difficulty, not a serious premature ejaculation problem. I saw them weekly for 3 times and then every 3 weeks for 4 months. At the end of therapy, Jane was orgasmic, Bill was choosing when to ejaculate and lasting for at least 5 minutes of intercourse. Jane, an anxiety-ridden obsessional person, became depressed for 2 weeks in response to my request that she tell me about her parent's marriage. Bill never wavered in his devotion and patience, even when her accusations were wildly unrealistic. His ability to help her with her worries gave him a sense of purpose that had been missing in his celibate life. With my steady encouragement, Jane directed Bill how to move during intercourse for her pleasure without crying that he did not know how to do it, without imagining that they would not have a good sex life, or that she should give him up before he hurts her. Bill was an eager student, had thick skin, and knew "in my heart that Jane doesn't mean half the things she says to me." She left her conjoint psychotherapy happy and was optimistic about Bill's trustworthiness and the safety of marrying him. They set a date.

THE TYPICAL DRAMA AMONG OLDER COUPLES

The sexual equilibrium is not just a concept that is useful for new couples. Its applicability persists throughout the life cycle. Balance of sexual capacities and regard are always important issues. When capacities are compatible and regard remains positive, their subtle interplays are not even noticed.

Anxiety about the drama of the formation of a new sexual equilibrium is palpable regardless of the age of the participants. Most of us worry if we will be pleasing to our new partners, whether we are 25 or 75 years of age.

As men and women move into their 60s, it is often apparent to them that their sexual capacities are not what they used to be. Women often have slower, less copious lubrication, shorter orgasms, and feel biologic drive less frequently. Men have comparable problems. Their arousal is less efficient and less dependable. Their biologic drive frequency and intensity are diminished. Orgasmic attainment is more work and invariably is not reached. Typically, it is the man who gives out first and withdraws from sexual activity. It is his attitude toward himself that ends and that renders their sexual equilibrium asexual. Here we have a reversal of the experience of young couples, where the woman's regard has the potential to shut down the young couple's sexual life. Among old couples, it is far more frequent that the man's negative regard for himself is the key factor in causing a cessation of sexual activity. He thinks destructive thoughts, such as "I can no longer get the job done." "Why humiliate myself?" "I am over the hill, I am impotent." "Old age is taking its toll on me already!"

These ideas arise in response to penile unreliability. Rather than using his reliable hands and mouth, he develops a dread of intercourse failure and avoids sexual activity, often without a word to his wife. This is not the only possible solution to the problem of diminishing sexual capacities.

> Seventy-one-year-old Donald had a car accident that rendered him briefly unconscious. His hospital stay was complicated by pneumonia. He resumed his active semiretirement after a month's recuperation. He fully recovered except for his potency. No organic etiology could be identified for his inability to obtain more than a floppy erection. A nocturnal tumescence test revealed no erections. Psychologically, he was happy, free of other symptoms, and had an intimate faithful marriage. Throughout his 8 months of impotence, he and his wife of 47 years continued to make love weekly, to attain orgasms, and to enjoy their relationship. "I guess my intercourse life is over. My sex life is not!"
>
> Donald had expected that he would lose his potency someday. He did not seem anxious about his deficiency and experienced little performance worry. "I have had and continue to have a good life." Donald preferred potency to his current state, but he chose not to have one of the modern techniques for restoring erections. "We are still doing fine. I just came in to see whether there was something I was missing in my appraisal of the situation."

The sexual developmental task of older couples is to keep the pleasure going. Donald and his wife illustrate that this is possible despite the very condition that is viewed by many others as the sufficient reason to stop all sexual behavior.

SUMMARY

The sexual equilibrium is the most misunderstood influence on our sexual lives. Sexual behavior with a partner takes place in an arena referred to as the *sexual equilibrium.* Two processes transpire and are balanced within it: the interaction of sexual components and the perception of partner regard. These processes occur throughout the life cycle. When two people make love, their individual sexual capacities and style interact and are sensed and reacted to by the partner. This process generates positive or negative regard. Positive regard from partner is crucial to the ability to relax and become lost in sensual expression. Negative regard from the partner typically induces an increase in self-consciousness that leads to sexual inhibition and harsh attitudes toward the self and the partner.

In newly formed couples, the developmental task is to establish a sexual equilibrium that affords both partners the opportunity to realize intense arousal and orgasmic attainment. The misery that derives from harsh partner regard sows the seeds for the premature cessation of sexual life. Although negative regard from the partner remains a danger to the continuation of sexual activity at all ages, older couples' sexual lives often end abruptly because of one person's harsh, defensive attitude toward the self.

It is clinically apparent that the same sexual conditions that create misery in some couples are present in happily adjusted couples. Positive regard of the partner and her or his sexual capacities is the key to such happiness. Unfortunately, in our rush to understand sexual life in nonsexual terms, clinicians can overlook the subtle, rapid, simultaneous exchange of attitude that can dampen a couple's sexual potential.

REFERENCES

1. Levine, SB: *Sex Is Not Simple.* Columbus, Ohio, Psychology Publications, 1989.
2. Bergler E: *Divorce Won't Help.* New York, Harper, 1948.
3. Masters WH, Johnson V: *Human Sexual Inadequacy.* Boston, Little, Brown, 1970.

CHAPTER 8

Helping Men to Control Ejaculation

Young and middle-aged men often long to lengthen the duration of their sexual intercourse experiences. Clinicians can help—sometimes—and in ways that do not require long-term therapy.

THE DISORDER OF PREMATURE EJACULATION

There must be a disorder called premature ejaculation. It is listed in the DSM-IV.[1] Throughout this century, numerous professional papers have been published on this topic. In several surveys, in Europe and in the United States, up to 40% of men acknowledge that they have the problem.[2,3] Many women feel that their sexual opportunities are limited by their partner's quick ejaculation. Treatments, reputed to be highly efficacious, exist and are widely promulgated as the correct approach to the problem.[4] But could premature ejaculation be an illusion?

Well, rapid ejaculation exists. Ejaculation before the couple desires it exists. Uncontrollability of the moment of orgasm also exists. It is just that labeling these phenomena with a diagnosis of premature ejaculation makes me uncomfortable. People seek out clinicians for help with this pattern and arrive with their self-diagnosis on their tongues. Men wear these diagnoses as badges of disgrace. I am uneasy because sometimes people reach the wrong conclusions about themselves.

Too many times, for example, I have met a naive couple in a marriage lacking in warmth and civility with this chief complaint. Too many times I have met frightened, uncomfortable sexual novices who unnecessarily complicate their lives with this label. I have also met frightened women without the capacity to tolerate their own sexual arousal, who have convinced themselves and their husbands that the problem is premature ejaculation. As a result of these and other experiences with the same complaint, I now view rapid ejaculation less as a diagnosis and more as an invitation to consider how the patient fits into the differential diagnosis.

Premature ejaculation is a heterosexual disorder of sexual physiology characterized by an untameably low threshold for the reflex sequence of orgasm. This physiological stubbornness allows the man to move through the phase of sexual arousal too fast. This persistent inability to experience a sense of control over the initiation of orgasm typically creates brief intravaginal latency times ranging from immediate to less than half a minute. Time alone can be a misleading indicator of the disorder, however. The heart of the diagnosis is the man's inability to influence his arousal responses to the sensations of physical intimacy. Whereas most men ejaculate sometimes before they wish to, the diagnosis of premature ejaculation requires persistence.

Differential Diagnosis

The other items on the differential diagnosis that must be given serious consideration before a clinician agrees with the man's diagnosis of premature ejaculation are:

1. Sexual inexperience
2. New problematic sexual equilibrium
3. High expectations for intravaginal containment time
4. Performance anxiety stimulated by fear of losing the partner
5. An intensely uncomfortable sexual partner
6. Deceitful proclamation of self-blame as a cover for his infidelity
7. Partner's blame of the man for sexual inadequacy as a cover for her infidelity
8. Fear of an adverse health event during intercourse

These items are not discrete from one another. They have several vital emotional forces in common: anxiety about intravaginal performance; notions of how sexual relations ought to be for each partner; the aspiration that the couple's sexual equilibrium will provide a mutually nurturant connection; and the man's basic responsibility for his partner's sexual happiness. It appears that a man's anxieties about his contribution to the sexual equilibrium may lower the ejaculatory threshold or keep it from its natural evolution to a higher level.

WHERE HAVE ALL THE SIMPLE CASES GONE?

Clinicians did not always have this differential diagnosis. Men who said they had premature ejaculation had premature ejaculation. A clinical caveat—a warning not to be this naive—is in order. Simple cases of premature ejaculation, the kind all clinicians long to treat with little more than the sensate focus and the stop–start technique, are now so difficult to find that experienced clinicians often whimsically ask, "Where did all the premature ejaculation go?" I have heard the question answered in three ways: we cured them all in the early days; men who would be the new simple cases now cure themselves by reading; the early easy cases were an artifact of our limited understanding of the complexity of people's sexual lives.

Today, we are largely left with complicated cases—persistent ones that have not improved with self-help techniques and those that are described in the differential diagnosis list. Simple cases must exist in the population because people are constantly coming of age and forming new sexual equilibriums. Premature ejaculation may not be in vogue any longer as a reason to seek help. In the early 1970s, the media gave much attention to this problem, because spectacular treatment results had just been reported by Masters and Johnson.[5] Today, more complicated matters, such as desire disorders, attract the attention.

MODERN TREATMENT HISTORY

Masters and Johnson's Format for Treatment

Modern treatment of premature ejaculation begins with Masters and Johnson, even though one of the methods they used, the Semans squeeze technique, was devised earlier.[6] Working during the 1960s, Masters and Johnson devised a general approach to sexual dysfunction called *sensate focus* into which they integrated the Semans squeeze technique for premature ejaculation. They published the best treatment results for this dysfunction that have ever been demonstrated: After a 5-year follow-up of 196 couples, 98% were recovered.

It is important to understand how this was possible, since these rates are not attained for most treatable psychiatric problems—then or now. Paying in advance, only couples came to the Masters and Johnson offices daily for up to 2 weeks for treatment. They left home, jobs, and children and stayed at a nearby hotel. After a thorough history taking, they were instructed in sensate focus exercises:

1. Day One Sensate Focus: taking turns giving and receiving pleasure without involving breasts or genitals.
2. Day Two Sensate Focus: taking turns giving and receiving pleasure involving the breasts.
3. Day Three Sensate Focus: taking turns giving and receiving pleasure involving breasts and each partner's genitals. This included learning how to stimulate the clitoris, vulva, and vagina in order to

help women attain orgasm and how to stimulate the penis in order to help men control the moment of their orgasm.

4. Day Four Sensate Focus: adding intercourse to the repertoire; first, quiet containment in the vagina, then female-governed movements, and finally, male-governed movements.

These steps were not necessarily taken on successive days. When a couple mastered the challenges of Day One Sensate Focus, they were given the Day Two instructions. If they required a week of visits to relax and take turns giving pleasure and concentrating on sensation when they were receiving pleasure, they took a week. It often took time to master these pleasant-sounding exercises because people resisted doing them or had many interfering feelings about being sensuous together. The male–female therapy team spent time helping the couple to understand their feelings, to deal with their hesitations, and to teach them the principles of good sexual functioning.

When the couple was judged to be ready for penile stimulation, the woman was instructed to sit between the legs of her prone, hands-to-the-side husband and to caress his erection. His role was to lie quietly feeling his sensations. His only other responsibility was to signal his partner when he felt his excitation rise to the point where he would ejaculate if she caressed him a few times more. At that point, she squeezed the glans penis firmly between her thumb and first two fingers. This action did not hurt the man; it only interrupted his rising excitation. The couple would relax for a half a minute or so and she would repeat the penile caressing. He would signal again when he was getting close to orgasm. She would squeeze and they would rest again. Usually, this had a wonderful effect on the couple because they could see that already he was receiving more stimulation than ever before and he was not ejaculating.

When the therapist team decided they could progress to intercourse, the couple was instructed to use the woman-on-top position, sitting, so that she could do with her vagina what she previously did with her hand— that is, stimulate his penis and, with his help, monitor his excitation. The first penile-vaginal intercourse was to be containment without motion. If he felt his excitation rising, he signaled her. She withdrew his penis enough to squeeze the glans. They rested, inserted again until quiet containment in the vagina no longer created uncontrollable excitation. When this was accomplished, the woman was instructed to slowly begin thrusting. She would stop anytime he requested for a squeeze of the glans. When female thrusting was mastered, the couple was instructed to move onto male thrusting.

In this manner, the couple learned to pay attention to both of their bodies during foreplay, to communicate during genital stimulation about his excitement, and to cooperate during intercourse. The couple, now working as a team, had a new freedom. The man lost his badge of dishonor and the woman often became more excited during her ministering to her husband than she ever did before. Some women had orgasms for the first time in their lives. The couple went home happy, grateful, and continued to provide positive feedback during their therapist's follow-up phone calls.

Patient selection factors were very important to Masters and Johnson's results. The patients were all motivated and financially able to come to St. Louis for 2 weeks of therapy. They were also on a vacation of sorts with an expectation of almost daily sexual homework assignments. Ordinary stresses of life were lifted. The therapists' enthusiasm was high. They were conducting a clinical experiment that seemed to show from the beginning that it could revolutionize the way we thought about sex and its problems.

It is hard to imagine today how little information was available during the 1960s about human sexuality. The culture was still shrouded in darkness. Masters and Johnson therapy teams provided illuminating principles that freed many people from ignorance and culturally induced restraint. They emphasized that sexual pleasure was natural—normal—and that inhibition was acquired and could be removed. They not only gave permission to the couple to enjoy themselves, but they also taught them how to use their bodies for their individual and mutual pleasure without performance anxieties. These patient, therapist, and cultural factors are ideal conditions for improvement.

Kaplan's Modifications

In the early 1970s, Helen Singer Kaplan simplified the treatment of these couples by suggesting that, rather than squeezing the glans, the couple should just stop what they are doing. This came to be known as the *stop–start technique.*[7] Kaplan also put the work of Masters and Johnson in a dynamic language that the mental health professionals could understand and demonstrated that couples could be seen much less frequently. Her formulations allowed "sex therapy" to be integrated into individual, couples, and group psychotherapy formats. She delineated how to recognize and work with the resistances to sensate focus recommendations.

Kaplan agreed with Masters and Johnson that premature ejaculation was relatively simple to treat. Their syntheses suggested that the previously predominant ideal that the premature ejaculation was a neurotic symptom that was due to unconscious conflict was either wrong or, if correct, did not require the standard treatment for unconscious difficulties. Masters and Johnson pointed to the lack of evidence to support the notion that individual psychotherapy had ever demonstrated that it was effective for this dysfunction. By the middle 1970s, it was clear that a revolution in therapy had occurred.

Treatment Works, but . . .

The behavioral treatment of premature ejaculation requires the therapist to teach the man to monitor his penile sensations, signal his partner, and practice his homework assignments until this task of prolonging intravaginal containment time is accomplished. Young clinicians are often eager to teach these techniques because they work. In doing so, the therapy simultaneously helps the patient's sex life and the therapist's professional identity as competent.

Choosing the right patient and selecting the correct time for using the technique are now the challenge. Before we consider these vital matters, I want to return in more depth to the male experience as a sexual partner because this information is sufficient to help some men overcome their rapid ejaculation. Some men with rapid ejaculation do not need treatment *per se,* rather, they only require education about the nature of ejaculatory control.

THE PASSION–CONTROL DILEMMA

Penile stimulation by hand, mouth, or vagina presents a man with a dilemma. The more he feels the exquisite sensations provided for him by his partner, the more aroused he becomes, and the closer he gets to orgasm, which ends his pleasure. During intercourse, for instance, the man has a choice: he can give in to his escalating pleasure, feel the passion, and burst into orgasm or he can opt for control, prolong intercourse, and have a quieter orgasm. Most men begin their sexual lives trying to do both. They attempt to make their passionate feelings last longer.

They cannot accomplish their goal for the simple reason that passion and control are opposites. There is an inherent dichotomy between passion and control. Passion is by its nature brief but intense; control is by its nature cool. No one escapes the grip of the passion–control dilemma. At any given moment a man can either select passion or control. The compromise that seems compatible with being a thoughtful, able sexual partner is to keep the movements of intercourse to a controllable pleasure until the decision is made to be swept away with a brief passionate run to orgasm. This is what the premature ejaculator cannot do—that is, keep his arousal to a low level in the vagina under most circumstances. The premature ejaculator does not have an option. Passion initially overwhelms him. Rather than viewing this as a lovely testimony to the power of intimacy to move him, he attributes it to his inadequacy and begins to be anxious about intercourse. A dangerous cycle begins because anxiety can keep the ejaculatory threshold low. A few misinterpreted passionate experiences and he is vulnerable to being trapped.

The Partner's Influence

The clinical problem is that the resolution of the passion–control dilemma is influenced by the partner. If a partner is one of the rare few who can consistently attain orgasm in response to the man's in-and-out thrusting movements, the man will have little need to create a strategy for control. He does not have to be nervous about when he reaches orgasm; he can just enjoy the experience. Soon, he will last longer in the vagina.

The search for a control strategy stems from the vast majority of women who do not find male-centered thrusting to be their best mode of arousal. One of the principles of the sexual equilibrium is that the sexual fate of one person is tied to the capacities and attitudes of the partner. The search for a control strategy is not a calm pursuit for most men. Desperation can quickly set in. The partner may calm or exacerbate his concerns about how he ought to be able to perform during intercourse. Unless the woman is particularly calming, the man begins to search for mental tricks to delay ejaculation.

Tricks for Prolonging Intercourse

The most commonly employed trick by men with rapid ejaculation is to think about something else during lovemaking, especially during intercourse. It may be sports, business, a horrifying scene from his life, nonsense syllables—anything that will take him away from his arousal. When this fails, condoms, preliminary masturbation to orgasm, or local anesthetics may be tried. Perhaps these tricks work for some men, but they have failed among those who become patients.

Clinicians have different suggestions for prolonging intercourse which are based on encouraging the man to be there emotionally for lovemaking rather than retreating from its sensations. Clinicians recognize that the mechanics of intercourse are important to the timing of ejaculation. The man may avoid passion at first by simply being still in the vagina. This was Masters and Johnson's recommendation for how to resume intercourse and gain ejaculatory control. The rapid rise of excitation may also be avoided by pacing the thrusting slowly or by having his partner move in a manner that does not create friction along the shaft of the penis. The woman-on-top position is often the best one to use in order to delay the escalation of male arousal. It provides weight constraints to the man's pelvic movements and encourages him to avoid movements that stimulate the shaft of the penis. This position simultaneously allows the woman the freedom to move her body along the head-to-toe horizontal plane rather than up and down on the penile shaft. Such motion, when freely engaged in, typically leads the woman to orgasm because it provides both the sensations of deep penile containment and intense clitoral stimulation.

When the man decides to opt for a passionate run to orgasm, he usually thrusts in and out of the vagina along the shaft of his penis at an increasing pace. The vagina is ideally suited to provide stimulation because it tends to fit his penis like a glove, maximizing friction. Typically, when the man feels the first sensations of orgasm, he pushes his penis deeply into the vagina and becomes still in order to perceive orgasm without distraction. When a man ejaculates while attempting to bring his partner to orgasm, he typically does not stop thrusting. As a result, he distracts himself from the sensations of orgasm. Many men who seek help for premature ejaculation describe muted and even pleasureless orgasms during intercourse.

THE TACTICAL ERRORS OF MEN
WITH PREMATURE EJACULATION

Clinicians need to know that men who have no ability to control their arousal within the vagina consistently make three errors. The first error is that they have a tactical plan for lovemaking—to minimize sexual arousal at all costs! We know this plan exists because they often instruct their partners not to touch the penis in stimulating ways and they avoid touching their partners in ways that excite them. Their partners' arousal is a problem for them because it is contagious—they find themselves further aroused. This tactic backfires badly. By controlling spontaneity and the possibility of arousal during foreplay, they trap themselves as poor lovers. They then miss the point by a wide margin by attributing their failures as lovers to their premature ejaculation. In reality, they are poor lovers because of the destructive rules they impose on lovemaking.

While these men are concentrating on not getting too excited during foreplay, they are unavailable to pay any attention to their sensations. When they begin intercourse, they are so anxious about when they will ejaculate that they ignore their sensations and miss the buildup of arousal. They often are deliberately trying to think about other matters during lovemaking. This avoidance of sensation is their second error. Masters and Johnson's therapeutic strategy was centered on enabling them to learn how to pay attention to sensations first outside, then inside, the vagina.

The third tactical error takes place when orgasm occurs. These men spoil the intensity of their orgasm by thrusting during it or by apologizing for its occurrence immediately after ejaculation. The apology follows from their worry that they will ejaculate too fast, their frustration caused by yet another failure, and their shame over their masculine inadequacy. These affect-laden processes reach a peak at the 2- to 4-second stage of ejaculatory inevitability prior to ejaculation. Orgasm, which has a great potential for intense pleasure, has frustration and shame superimposed on it by them. They think or say, "Oh shit!" or "I'm sorry" at the moment their partners are scrambling to increase their own arousal. The men begin to talk, to apologize at a time when listening to an apology is not what the partners had in mind. After several repetitions of the interfering apology, partners are often crying, thinking of ways of torturing and murdering their partners, or writing off the possibilities of mutual pleasure.

These errors tell us that the premature ejaculator has not yet figured out an important principle of sexual functioning: The best way to increase the capacity to sustain a high level of arousal without ejaculation is to experience sexual intensity. The nervous system accommodates to stimulation by raising the threshold for the ejaculatory reflex. This is how young, rapidly ejaculating men eventually improve and how sensate focus with the squeeze or the stop–start technique operates. On their own, without the benefit of the insights of the pioneers of sex therapy, men reach the opposite conclusion. Their tactic to avoid excitement during lovemaking is logical to them because arousal seems to be the problem. What happens, sadly, is that these men trap themselves in their anxious, threshold-lowering behavior by removing themselves from the very processes that enable other men to gain ejaculatory control.

The cornerstone of modern therapy for men with rapid ejaculation is to instruct and enable them to tolerate progressively increasing sexual intensity. Premature ejaculators need to stop their concern over performance and begin to seek pleasure and intensity rather than control. They need to shift back toward passion on the passion–control spectrum. They must stop trying to think of other matters during lovemaking. They must no longer react to their orgasms with disappointment and apology. They must be available to feel every last muscular contraction of their orgasm and allow their partners to hear the vocalizations of their orgasm as it occurs.

We are now able to understand the common instructions given to a couple during therapy. The man is told that when orgasm occurs, whether it was sooner than he wanted it or not, he is to enjoy it. Apologies and apologetic thinking are to be banished. In their place, sounds of his orgastic pleasure are to be encouraged. He is permitted to ejaculate without moving in the vagina. The couple is informed that the purpose of these instructions is not only to increase the pleasure of his orgasm, but also to increase her pleasure over his orgasm.

The partner is helped to not consider her sexual opportunities over when his orgasm occurs. She is told that the length of detumescence is proportional to the degree of arousal throughout their lovemaking. She is taught how to move on his body for her pleasure, using whatever penile tumescence that remains, and is assured that a woman does not have to have a penis in her vagina to attain orgasm. Many heterosexual women have not considered that homosexual women can be orgasmic by moving against each other's pubic bone. The idea that a woman need not be dependent on his trusting of an erect penis for her sexual pleasure usually has two positive effects: she is freed from her sense of helpless dependence on him; and he visibly relaxes in the office and reports less worry about intercourse.

THREE CLUES ABOUT THE PHYSIOLOGY OF EJACULATION

The foregoing discussion of rapid ejaculation is consistent with the idea that its uncontrollability is a psychosocial learning disorder. Throughout this century, premature ejaculation has been considered a psychogenic dysfunction. Several observations provide cautions to this widespread assumption.

Age

Rapid ejaculation typically is a young man's normative problem. The prevalence of premature ejaculation is significantly higher among young men. Once premature ejaculation becomes well-established within a sexual equilibrium, however, it can last a lifetime. The typical ejaculatory pattern of older men is progressive difficulty in triggering off the orgasmic reflex. Something basically physiologic is occurring as men age. Youth often evidences a hair-trigger responsiveness to the warmth, wetness, friction, and symbolic meanings of the vagina. Men in middle life may think that they have finally mastered their rapid ejaculation—finally, they can choose passion or control. In older age, men begin to notice that it is sometimes difficult and sometimes impossible to attain orgasm. By the time most men are aware of this, they are already familiar with the fact that their refractory period—the time it takes after orgasm to become sufficiently aroused to maintain another erection—long ago lengthened from their youthful hour or so to at least several days. Older men may also observe that they may not be able to trigger off an orgasm when a long time has passed since their last sexual opportunity. This pattern is distinctly different from their youth.

That something important is occurring in the physiological substrate of sexual physiology is obvious. What is occurring is not. Sexual capacities decline with age, including the capacity to reach orgasm. These declines are not simply related to circulating testosterone levels. The sexual defect among aging men is far more subtle and clearly has yet to be discovered.

Whatever explains these ejaculation changes with advancing age will probably also explain why neither desire, arousal, or orgasm are exactly what they used to be.

The Premature Ejaculator and Age

There is one pertinent variation on the theme of sexual decline. Some men with premature ejaculation do not outgrow their condition with advancing age. They retain their lifelong pattern of rapid ejaculation in the vagina regardless of their age until erectile dysfunction becomes the limiting factor for intercourse. Even then, some premature ejaculators reach orgasm quickly near the vagina with a semiflaccid penis. This seeming invulnerability to the sexual consequences of age on orgasm suggests two possible explanations: either premature ejaculators are different physiologically or the psychology that generates this persistent symptom is more powerful than the physiological decrements of time. Beatrice's experience provides an illustrative example of the timelessness of some premature ejaculation.

"It has been a feast after years of famine for me," a 72-year-old, recently retired, energetic, healthy lawyer explained. "I have met two wonderful men both in their early seventies. The one I love the most, and would marry in a flash, is a remarkably sensitive lover but has trouble maintaining an erection. I really don't care that much, I have wonderful orgasms with him and I try to show him all the time how pleased I am just to be with him. The trouble is that he is elusive and frightened to love me.

"The other, who wants to marry me and cannot stop telling me and the world how much he loves me, comes fast all the time. It is still fun being with him, he is so eager and excited. I'm gently trying to teach him to slow down on everything and take his time, but he is used to quick unhappy intercourse with his ex-wife. He is embarrassed about his ejaculation but pleased as punch about his erections.

Serotonergic Uptake Inhibitors

In the last few years, two drugs, fluoxitane (Prozac) and clomipramine (Anafranil), have been approved for use and become widely prescribed by psychiatrists in the United States. Prozac is primarily used as an antidepressant, whereas Anafranil, also an antidepressant, is used primarily as a treatment for obsessive-compulsive disorder. Each drug is a postsynaptic serotonin-uptake inhibitor, meaning that each increases the concentration of this neurotransmitter at key synapses in the nervous system. This is of great interest to the treatment of sexual disorders because the serotonin system has long been suggested to play a dampening role in human sexual expression.

More importantly for the treatment of premature ejaculation, patients taking standard doses of these drugs often complain that they have difficulty ejaculating. While these observations are still anecdotal, they are so widely reported that some clinicians have begun to use the drugs—especially clomipramine—as a treatment for uncontrollable ejaculation. Clomipramine is used because ejaculation is delayed at doses that are subtherapeutic for obsessive-compulsive symptoms. The dose of fluoxitane that may slow ejaculation is the same as the therapeutic dose and is likely to lead to sleep difficulties.

Assalian has reported on 12 men who failed to improve with the standard behavioral treatment protocol for premature ejaculation.[8] Each demonstrated dramatic, quick improvement of intravaginal latency to orgasm times on doses of clomipramine between 25 and 75 mg daily. These observations are preliminary. Single or double-blind treatment protocols have not been published. It is possible that expectancy effects are producing the results. Nonetheless, I, too, have had the clinical experience of providing a low dose of clomipramine to men who have unsuccessfully tried to overcome their rapid ejaculatory patterns. These experiences have been so positive, dose-related, and predictable that it is hard not to be enthusiastic that these drugs may be an answer for men whose ejaculatory threshold is not influenced by the behavioral principles that allow most men to overcome their initially physiologic stubbornness. In keeping with the normal effects of age on ejaculation, young men I have treated with clomipramine require more drug than those in their sixties. This may reflect changes in absorption and metabolic degradation with age as well as the sensitivity of the sexual physiological system. Stay acquainted with the clinical science literature, because scientifically acceptable studies will probably soon appear.

These three observations—the decrement of rapid ejaculation with time, the persistence of premature ejaculation in some men, and the promise of a medication to raise the threshold of orgasm—suggest to me that the psychogenic disorder of premature ejaculation may be a mixture of biologic, social, and psychological vulnerabilities.

USING THE DIFFERENTIAL DIAGNOSIS

Sexual Inexperience

Men beginning their heterosexual experience do not usually seek help for rapid ejaculation. Clinicians may hear about their pattern if they or their partner are in therapy for some other matter. Rapid ejaculation should not surprise anyone, however. Sexual intercourse is an important rite of passage about which young men worry. The long-imagined-but-not-yet-experienced woman's body can be so exciting that the young man ejaculates or nearly ejaculates even before intercourse. Excitement over a woman's body may last a lifetime but soon the novelty, the anxiety, and the overwhelming sensations of physical intimacy diminish. It is this evolution that is interfered with in the men who become premature ejaculators.

A Problematic New Sexual Equilibrium

In the early days of treating men and their partners for premature ejaculation with the new sex therapy treatment protocol, we would often encounter a partner who resisted carrying out the therapeutic suggestions. She would pleasantly agree to do the homework assignment, but would avoid doing it or would do it half-heartedly. This experience does not occur as often today because we take a better history of the woman's comfort with her sexuality. We are highly interested in her arousal capacities and orgasmic patterns. We used to assume that the anorgasmic wives of premature ejaculators were victims of their husbands' dysfunctions. Now, we are more cognizant of the possibility that the woman and the man are equally uncomfortable about sexual experiences. We have come to realize that the female partner may need as much attention, education, encouragement, and opportunity to articulate her fears as her rapidly ejaculating partner. The correct diagnostic focus is on the sexual equilibrium rather than on the man or the woman. Anxious beginners require therapeutic optimism, a calm perspective about the universality of sexual discomfort, and sometimes specific instructions about how to teach each other. I am often openly skeptical about revealing their diagnosis to them, preferring a wait-and-see attitude. When couples are approached together with calm optimism, one partner may continue to be unable to cooperate with the sexual opportunities. At this point, individual sessions are often started to help the person understand the motives for not cooperating with therapy. During the 1970s, many of the treatments for male-centered dysfunctions abruptly ended with neither the man nor his wife receiving significant help. We simply did not understand the nature of the resistance.

Unrealistic Expectations for the Duration of Intercourse

All clinicians are occasionally surprised by people's expectations for their sexual experience. A man or a couple seeking help for premature ejaculation may shock the therapist by reporting that their intravaginal latency is only 5 minutes of intense male-on-top thrusting, for example. It is "premature" because it used to be much longer; he cannot bring his partner to orgasm, or he has believed the stories told by others about their lengthy periods of intercourse. Kinsey and his colleagues asked a large sample of men how long their intercourses lasted. The majority reported less than 2 minutes.[9]

Some substance-abusing men discover that they have less intravaginal thrusting capacities when they are sober and off their central nervous system (CNS)-acting drugs. The intravaginal time may be the most important concern of the patient, but the clinician's focus on the history and the reasons for the expectation often quickly illuminates the man's circumstances. The evaluation may calm the man. The loss of anxiety may improve his intravaginal time or help him to stop clocking the time of his intercourses.

Some men have excellent ejaculatory control from the beginning of their partner sexual experiences. Very soon they may be able to have intercourse for as long as they like. When they become anxious, their concerns about premature ejaculation may not be taken seriously by the clinician because they can now last only 5 minutes. The man is sincere, the clinician thinks he is exaggerating. Time, by itself, can be a misleading indicator of the diagnosis.

Performance Anxiety Stimulated by Fear of Losing the Partner

A large minority of men seeking help for premature ejaculation are, in fact, in a marital or relationship crisis. They may never have outgrown their early rapid ejaculation entirely, but their fears of abandonment are now part of their emotional experience during lovemaking. Often, these fears are superimposed on his angry feelings toward his partner during intercourse prior to her threats of leaving. The therapist should not undertake a treatment for premature ejaculation in the face of such a crisis. The couple should be helped to deal with the larger issues in their life first. Once they decide to deal with their basic interactional problems and reestablish their commitment to remain together, then, if the rapid ejaculation is still present, they can attend to the ejaculatory problem.

Male Deceit

Sometimes a man experiences rapid ejaculation with his wife, but not with his lover. His wife, who is unaware of his extramarital experiences, pleads that they seek help for the premature ejaculation. He knows he is not a premature ejaculator, but he prefers to have her think that he is in order to keep her from wanting to make love with him. These are delicate situations. Clinicians must respect people's confidential disclosures, yet, must not lie to the spouse to protect the other. Typically, the therapist offers the man several options: to discuss the truth as a couple, to have individual sessions with the man, or to no longer meet since the therapist cannot in good faith participate in the deception of the wife. If the wife wants individual sessions, the therapist needs to carefully wait while she discovers the truths of her marriage. I often think that rapid ejaculation by a man with a regularly cheated-upon wife indicates that it is a conscious or nearly conscious expression of his disdain, a cover for his deceit, and a rationalization of doing his marital duty.

Female Deceit

Similar principles govern the management of triangulated couples regardless of the gender of the deceiver. It is ethically untenable for the therapist to willfully participate in the perpetuation of a lie. It not only can backfire on the therapist, but it can prove highly destructive to both members of the couple. Therapy requires honesty to realize its full potential. Often when dishonesty is basic to the proceedings, no lasting therapeutic gains are made.

Health Concerns

Men commonly develop rapid ejaculation after a myocardial infarction. Usually, it is not difficult for the therapist to perceive that the man is protecting himself from his fears of an arrhythmia, chest pain, or sudden death. Similarly, a man can be anxious about the new health status of his wife and get intercourse over with quickly in order to spare her adverse consequences or to protect himself. Some people worry that cancer is contagious through intercourse, for example. Other men may develop premature ejaculation as a way of limiting the possibility that their wives may become short of breath. Since serious diseases increase with advancing age, clinicians should be curious about any new rapid-ejaculation patterns that develop around a change in health status of either partner.

PSYCHOTHERAPY AND RAPID EJACULATION

Men with rapid ejaculation still seek individual psychoanalytically oriented psychotherapy for these sexual problems. Clinicians evaluating couples with this complaint still choose to see one partner in a talking therapy rather than using a couples' behavioral therapy format. These are not necessarily signs of therapeutic incompetence or ideologic stubbornness. Premature ejaculation seems quite capable of deriving from the hidden meanings of the vagina to men. Their nervousness during intercourse or about their competence as lovers may sometimes be explained by their fears of closeness to women. I learned this lesson very early in my attempt to gain experience with the Masters and Johnson format.

A psychoanalyst referred a man for treatment of premature ejaculation that he had been seeing off and on for 20 years. This obsessive-compulsive 58-year-old never impotent bachelor brought a cooperative, kind partner, a friend of many years, with whom he had sexual intercourse on occasion. As I explained the plans for treatment, he blanched and said that he thought he was going to be impotent. Throughout our attempt to work as a couple with behavioral techniques, he never could obtain an erection. After 7 sessions, it had become clear to all three of us that further therapy for premature ejaculation was not wise. At a 1-month follow-up visit, he reported that he became potent again immediately after we stopped our weekly meetings but that his 10-second and best intercourse capacity remained.

More recently, a 38-year-old married man attained ejaculatory control for the first time in his life after 4 months of weekly talking psychotherapy. He spent little time during his therapy talking about this symptom, although this was why he sought help. Instead, he spent most hours telling me stories about his mother's manipulative, controlling, demeaning style of loving him. His far fewer stories of his deceased father were also focused on the dangerousness of being close to him and his sadness at not having spent more time with him. He worked hard at understanding what had happened to him, wondering what feelings he was entitled to and what were the signs that he was an ungrateful bad son. I did not have to suggest that his fears of reencountering the double-binding powers of his mother in sexual intimacy with his wife kept him anxious about initiating intercourse and quick in his response to being in the vagina. I did not have to explain that the vagina had become a symbol of the dangers of closeness to his mother. The more this bright man talked, the more he could feel and see that his wife was victimized by his maternal transference. The frequency of intercourse went from once or twice a month to weekly and his estimated intravaginal latency increased from 10–30 seconds to 3 to 4 minutes. Apparently, he could not use the information about overcoming premature ejaculation he had read in books until he had a chance to discuss his conflicts, memories, and coping strategies about his mother.

SUMMARY

Learning how to maintain arousal in the vagina without triggering orgasm is a highly valued developmental goal for many heterosexual men. In surveys, up to 40% of men depict themselves as having premature ejaculation. Clinicians need to be prudent in selecting men for the behavioral treatment of this condition. Effective treatment requires the wholehearted cooperation of two people. Some men can be helped by brief discussions about their sexual situations, while others are participants in compromised relationships that preclude successful direct treatment of the untameable ejaculation. Two antidepressants, fluoxetane and clomipramine, appear to offer hope to men who do not respond to behavioral interventions. Although therapists should not expect that psycho-dynamic psychotherapy can enable ejaculatory control in a large percent-age of men, it is still used because of relationship situations and when men want to speak in private about their developmentally acquired fears about sexual closeness. When rapid ejaculation is considered more of a develop-mental task to be mastered and less of a disorder that requires a specific treatment, it is possible to be helpful to various men who have concerns about the conduct of intercourse. This requires, however, a sense of the differential diagnosis of rapid ejaculation and an awareness that the focus on the timing of ejaculation can be too narrow for effective clinical work.

REFERENCES

1. American Psychiatric Association: *Diagnostic and Statistical Manual of Mental Disorders*, ed. 4. Washington, DC, American Psychiatric Association, 1992.
2. Schein M, Zyzanski S, Levine SB, Dickman R, Alegomagno S: The frequency of sexual problems among family practice patients. *Family Practice Research Journal*, 1988; 7(3):122–134.
3. Bancroft J: *Human Sexuality and Its Problems*. Edinburgh, Churchill Livingstone, 1989.
4. Kaplan HS: *PE: Overcoming Premature Ejaculation*. New York, Brunner/Mazel, 1989.
5. Masters WH, Johnson V: *Human Sexual Inadequacy*. Boston, Little, Brown, 1970.
6. Semans JH: Premature ejaculation: A new approach. *Southern Medical Journal*, 1956; 49:353–357.
7. Kaplan HS: *The New Sex Therapy*. New York, Brunner/Mazel, 1974.
8. Assalian P: Is premature ejaculation psychogenic? Read before the Society for Sex Therapy and Research Meeting, Redondo Beach, California, March, 1991.
9. Kinsey AC, Pomeroy WB, Martin CE: *Sexual Behavior in the Human Male*. Philadelphia, WB Saunders, 1948.

CHAPTER 9

Helping Women to Become Orgasmic

Meager cultural encouragement for females to become adept at sexual expression explains some of the mystery of the elusive female orgasm. But more attention needs to be paid to the subtle roles that women play during partner sex.

BASIC ASSUMPTIONS

Three assumptions about women's orgasmic attainment guide my thinking about functional and dysfunctional sexual life. These ideas are not wholly scientifically proven and may never be. This is the way it is with much of our sexual knowledge—the work that clinicians do with individuals and the studies that sexologists do with groups often yield ideas about private sexual experience that stop short of certainty.

1. *Orgasmic attainment is frequently elusive.* The first notion is that orgasms with a partner are not quickly attained by many women. Women have to learn how to use their bodies during lovemaking in order to have orgasms. This fact stands in stark contrast with the common idea that orgasms either just happen or are delivered to the woman by her partner. The speed of learning how to become orgasmic varies considerably from woman to woman. Based on several studies, I imagine that at least 20% of women find orgasmic attainment with a partner elusive after they have made love twenty or so times. Orgasms are elusive for sexually inexperienced women, in part, because they are preoccupied with matters other than personal orgasmic pleasure during lovemaking, matters that produce interfering thoughts and distracting feelings. These feelings include: ensuring the partner's pleasure*; fear of what the partner will think

---

*This discussion has a heterosexual focus but the major principles being discussed here apply to homosexual relationships as well.

of her if she acts too excited; fear of her partner's reaction to her body; pregnancy worries; and the need to cope with the partner's anxiety about his orgasm. In addition, many young women have little idea of how to go about having an orgasm with a partner.

Orgasm with a partner is elusive in another sense; even among women who have learned how to reliably attain orgasms, orgasms are not invariably realized. Many concerns can distract a woman from the concentration on her pleasure that is necessary for attaining orgasm. It is a common experience for a sexually functional woman to have to explain to her partner that she did not have an orgasm and that it is all right. Men need this reassurance because it is apparent that women's experience with orgasm is not directly analogous to their own. Most young men are orgasmic each time they become excited with a partner. In the baseball vernacular, they bat one thousand. Very few orgasmic women attain orgasm during every sexual opportunity.

2. *Most women do not have orgasms through intercourse.* The second assumption is that about 50% of women who attain orgasms with their partners with some regularity are orgasmic during some form of intercourse. Although a minority of women are able to have orgasms in response to a variety of stimuli, women far more commonly use one means of attaining orgasm on most occasions. The usual means of orgasmic attainment with partners seem to be, in this order: manual stimulation of the clitoris, intercourse with the woman on top, intercourse with the man on top, oral stimulation, vibrator stimulation, the woman stimulating herself to orgasm in front of her partner.

3. *Every woman is biologically capable of orgasm.* The third assumption is that orgasmic attainment is normal, prewired into the nervous system, and within the biological capacities of nearly all physically healthy women. The fact that a large number of women do not realize their biologic potential is to be explained by social and psychological factors rather than biological ones. When more is known about the anatomic and physiologic components of orgasm, some anorgasmic females may be discovered to lack a necessary component, such as a paravertebral ganglion or a neurotransmitter. Until such evidence is accumulated, however, it seems prudent to assume that most women are biologically capable of orgasms.

Occasionally, however, a challenge to this assumption surfaces: such as orgasm is not important or "normal" for women. This argument, frequently presented in newspapers and magazines through surveys or write-in responses, emphasizes that women normally desire closeness, being held, and feeling their partner's attentive interest, rather than orgasm.

This idea is comforting for the nonorgasmic, but it seems to be dangerously specious. Nonorgasmic women have higher rates of dissatisfaction with sexual life.[1] The argument encourages anorgasmic women to lower their personal expectations and, therefore, their opportunities to learn how to attain orgasms. It also limits their understanding of the private world of other people's sexuality. Overall, the argument seems to be a disservice to enlightenment.

This argument, however, is just one example of the strong feelings that the topic of women's orgasm is capable of generating. Women's orgasm can quickly become a male–female political issue. Men are often accused of bringing their achievement-oriented sensibilities to the bedroom and spoiling the sublime relationship aspects of lovemaking by their emphasis on the orgasm above the pleasures of intimate caressing for its own sake. Furthermore, they are accused of introducing the woman to performance anxiety—that is, taking their own culturally driven male sexual insanity and bringing it, like a contagious disease, to the sexually developing young woman who then is made to feel defective or a failure because she cannot perform as he wants.

Men tend to view their sexual partners' consistent lack of orgasm as a sign that they are unloved, that they are inadequate in sexual technique, or that they possess a penis that is too small. A man who is part of a sexual equilibrium with a woman who is having difficulty attaining orgasm with him has to overcome these feelings. One of the destructive patterns used to obscure these feelings of unlovability and inadequacy is to cruelly blame the woman. She is called inadequate without ever directly acknowledging the meaning her orgasm has for him.

Such male behavior, of course, does little for the woman who is trying to figure out how to become orgasmic. Because she is interested in pleasing her partner, the woman soon becomes an anxious spectator during lovemaking rather than a sensual, focused participant. These dynamics—the spoken and unspoken thoughts and feelings of both partners—are enough to prevent many new sexual equilibria from providing emotional satisfaction from sexual behavior. They are also sufficient to induce some women to fake their orgasmic attainment.

Because I assume that orgasm is within the woman's biological capacity, I view her orgasmic attainment as her sexual developmental task. When she masters this task, she is free to move on to higher levels of sexual experience, such as having orgasms with different sources of stimulation, using more of her body with pleasure, focusing more efficiently on her sensations, and accepting her body without preoccupation with its flaws. When she cannot master orgasmic attainment with a partner, she is likely to lose some of her personal interest in sexual behavior and will not be able to grasp the experience of others without envy or the sense of personal inadequacy.

THE IMAGINARY EXPERIMENT

I would feel better about my three assumptions if a major, longitudinal, epidemiological study could be done to test each of them. The study would have to be prospective. It would have to have interview and objective measures done at reasonable intervals. "Regularly orgasmic" would have to be arbitrarily defined at a frequency level that made intuitive sense to a panel of female researchers. The sample size would have to be large and the subjects would have to be sufficiently multicultural to satisfy the requirement for ethnic diversity. The women and their partners would enter the study at the onset of their established sexual relationships and would have to remain subjects for 5 years.

This expensive study has not been done. But using the magic of my imagination, however, here are the results that I would expect: 10% of the women were regularly orgasmic from their first partner intimacies; 15% became regularly orgasmic within their first 10 experiences; 25% became orgasmic within their 11th to 25th experiences; 25% became orgasmic within 3 years of regular sexual opportunities; and 25% did not become regularly orgasmic during the study period. (We would examine similar data about ejaculatory control and discover similar findings.)

These five groups would be collapsed and relabeled as fast learners, moderately fast learners, slow learners, and the dysfunctional. We would then investigate the statistical relationships between these outcomes and the independent variables thought to be related to orgasmic attainment: adolescent masturbation to orgasm; age of onset of masturbation to orgasm; quality of relationship to each parent; preparation for menstruation; sexual identity; sexual knowledge; sibling order; religiosity; race; cultural and economic backgrounds; vacation; neuroticism; relationship health; childhood sexual abuse; and others.

The painstaking investigation of how well these variables predict orgasmic capacity, in my imagination, would show us that no one factor or one cluster of factors has an invariable predictive power. This would leave us with the idea that, while generally speaking, positive variables predicted faster and more frequent orgasmic attainment, some factors, either not actually measured or not validly measured in the study, explained most of the variance. The study would also show that, generally, women with the worst psychological backgrounds were heavily represented among the slow-learners and the dysfunctional.

Many actual small-scale studies have been done in an attempt to ascertain such information, but the power of science and the commitment of science funding are extremely limited in this area.[2] This imaginary study is my way of suggesting what is needed to establish facts from the widespread assumptions about women's orgasmic attainment. It is also a way of stating my assumptions with more direct clinical applicability: (1) orgasmic attainment is a personal sexual developmental task that women accomplish to varying degrees in their lives; and (2) orgasmic attainment problems are best explained by creating a dialogue over time with the woman about her thoughts, feelings, attitudes, and developmental experiences.

THE DIAGNOSIS OF ANORGASMIA

All problems of orgasmic attainment in women should not be quickly labeled as *disorders*. There are a variety of reasons for this sexual inability. Some are serious and require therapy. Others require only education and encouragement, and still others require attention to the woman's partner. Clinicians need to focus on the extent to which their patient's inability to attain an orgasm has been influenced by sexual inexperience, limited sexual learning opportunities prior to partner sexual behavior, as problematic partner, and the grip of unconscious psychic conflict. This is no easy clinical task.

Women who are diagnosed with the disorder of *anorgasmia* have failed to figure out how to attain orgasm after a long opportunity and now privately sense themselves as lacking the capacity. In this case study, Kate's psychological dilemma concerning orgasm is typical of women who are given this diagnosis.

Kate

At 31, Kate, a physically healthy, happily married mother of two pre-schoolers and a part-time mental health professional, is distressed at her inability to attain orgasm. She is aware of a personal paradox—she has a strong rational wish to have orgasms with her husband and seemingly stronger illogical notions that such intensity is for bad girls. "I am a good girl; your all-around nice person—well-organized, responsible, afraid of anyone's bad opinion of me, never in trouble, a good student."

Kate has sexual drive, although not nearly as much as her husband. She is receptive to his sexual advances and sometime initiates their sexual behavior. She generally has no problem being aroused and lubricates easily, but there have been times when she thought she deserved the diagnosis of inhibited sexual desire. She thinks she may have had a few orgasms with Peter in the months before marriage, but is not certain. Peter has been consistently willing to caress her genitals, have intercourse in any position, and engage in mouth–genital stimulation. She feels grossed out by cunnilingus and cannot understand why anyone would want to do such a thing.

During lovemaking, Kate becomes excited only to a certain point. After this pleasant level of arousal is attained, her mind wanders to thoughts about the many tasks she has to do. When she decides that she will not allow her mind to wander in this way, the experience is still suddenly over for her whenever she feels some deep sensual stirring.

Kate not only does not ever recall masturbating but has long felt that most girls and women do not do it either. She simply does not believe the facts to which she has been exposed during her undergraduate and graduate education. "It's ridiculous, I know, but the idea of it turns me off–proper people do not do such things."

Peter is sexually comfortable, encouraging, not pressuring, and feels that

Kate should seek help for herself because, while she is a good sexual partner, she does not seem to be able to stay with the pleasure during their weekly experiences.

During her third psychotherapy session, Kate points out that her orgasmic inhibition seems to be part of a larger pattern of avoiding emotional intensity. She fears that emotion, overexcitement from any source, will harm or change her. Being out of control is one of her worst fears. When pressed to explain the meaning of "out of control," she can only conclude that she means feeling too strongly about matters. In her work, she often hears herself telling others that their family interactions are too intense. She is good with ideas, writes notes a lot, and generally minimizes opportunities to be aroused in any way. "It is just the way I am, I have always been this way, I'm sure."

Kate has many friends and feels respect as a professional. She occasionally offers sexual counseling. "I either feel like a fraud telling women it is okay to enjoy themselves or I get jealous when I hear about the sexual capacities of my patients."

Psychiatric Attitudes toward Orgasmic Attainment

Professional attitudes toward women's orgasmic attainment have dramatically changed in recent decades. Prior to Masters and Johnson's 1970 book, *Human Sexual Inadequacy*,[3] the field of psychoanalysis had conceptual hegemony over the subject. Psychoanalytic theory promulgated three notions that persisted throughout most of this century: (1) women who were not orgasmic during intercourse, typically as a result of the man's active thrusting, were diagnosed as "frigid"; (2) women's pattern of relying upon clitoral stimulation for orgasmic attainment reflected psychosexual immaturity, neurosis, or frigidity, whereas the pattern of vaginal orgasmic attainment reflected psychosexual maturity or the authentic feminine response; (3) the deep and important causes of such sexual deficits were Oedipal guilt over continued longing for closeness to the father and penis envy.

Masters and Johnson's work on sexual physiology failed to confirm the psychoanalytic idea that there were separate vaginal and clitoral orgasms.[4] They stress that women's descriptions of different levels of emotional satisfaction, intensity of sensations, and preferences for types of stimulation to orgasm were explained by factors other than biological distinctions between types of orgasm. The objective physiological sameness of orgasm, no matter how it was stimulated or how it was perceived by the woman, led Masters and Johnson to dispute the psychological significance previously attributed to how orgasms were attained. Suddenly, the idea that a woman's general psychological maturity was reflected in her style of orgasmic attainment seemed irrational. Masters and Johnson repeatedly emphasized throughout the 1970s that orgasm was a similar physiological event from woman to woman—no matter how it was stimulated. Orgasm became known as a reflex triggered by the woman's muscular effort to augment her arousal from the lower plateau level to the higher reflex threshold level of arousal.

In their clinical work, Masters and Johnson referred to the problem of lack of female orgasm with a partner as "nonorgasmic return." Others quickly replaced this unharmonious phrase with a Latinized term "anorgasmia." During the 1970s, professionals all agreed that the cause of this problem was sociocultural and psychological. The understanding and resolution of these psychological factors, however, were not felt to require psychoanalysis.

Clinical research with young adult women by LoPiccolo and Lobitz,[5] Barbach,[6,7] and others[8] suggested that the psychological factors that kept a woman anorgasmic could be removed in 10-session, highly structured, educational, supportive groups that discussed the woman's genital anatomy, the role of the clitoris in arousal, masturbation, and techniques of intercourse with the woman's pleasure in mind. This work led to a semantic shift: women who have not yet acquired the ability to easily attain orgasm began being referred to as "preorgasmic." This new optimistic term conveyed the idea that it is only a matter of realizing the possibility and spending more time and energy doing some psychological work. The notion of the preorgasmic woman came out of the early energy of the Women's Movement. The adjective *anorgasmic,* on the other hand, implied that something is wrong with the woman. It seemed to be part of the medical tradition of men diagnosing women who were not equipped to please men.

With the politics of semantics set to one side, the initial impression that women who do not have orgasms with their partners were easily treatable was not readily confirmed by clinical experiences. Clinicians recognized that the new ideas were helpful but not always sufficient to budge a woman with tenaciously fearful attitudes. Critical review of the studies indicated that it was far easier to help "preorgasmic" women to become regularly orgasmic during masturbation than with a partner.[9] It was also appreciated that age was an important factor in response to these treatment techniques. The internal obstacles to the freedom to use the body for personal pleasure are far easier to overcome among college-aged women than their mothers. Twenty years of providing for the pleasures of the partner make the obstacles far harder to disrupt than when a woman is young, sexually inexperienced, and has the momentum of psychological development on her side.[10]

As with the well-defined technique for the treatment of premature ejaculation, the easy cases of orgasmic attainment seemed to have quickly disappeared from the clinical scene. The explanation for this is probably quite similar to that discussed in the last chapter. In addition, however, there have been cultural changes over the past two decades. Now orgasmic attainment for women is generally considered to be the norm. Culture is now providing permission for orgasm attainment and no longer looks to the institutions dominated by men to tell women how they should be.

THE SITUATIONS OF ORGASMIC ATTAINMENT

It is often said that orgasmic attainment is situational—orgasms are attainable under one set of social circumstances but not the one that the patient or partner thinks is appropriate. The frequent occurrence of situational anorgasmia means that the clinician must know the answers to the following questions before the woman's situation can be thought of as thoroughly assessed:

- Do you now have orgasms by self-stimulation during masturbation?
- Do you now have orgasms during hand stimulation of your genitals?
- Do you have orgasms during oral stimulation of your genitals?
- Do you have orgasms during vibratory stimulation of your genitals?
- Do you have orgasms with a partner other than the one I know about?
- Have you ever been able to have orgasms with a partner? If yes, how were they stimulated?
- Do you have orgasms if you use a particular type of fantasy? If yes, please describe the fantasy or fantasies.
- Under what conditions have you ever been orgasmic during your life? Dreams?

Not only do the answers to these questions elucidate the orgasmic pattern that underlies the chief complaint of "I cannot have an orgasm," they allow the history of the problem to emerge. Many apparently anorgasmic women are not actually anorgasmic. When the clinician hears, for example, that a woman is regularly orgasmic with her lover in several ways but is not able to attain orgasm with her husband, her problem is usually not considered in terms of anorgasmia, even though psychological forces at work make it impossible to have orgasms with her husband. In these "situational" problems, the diagnosis of anorgasmia is usually not a final one. Here, in outline form, are the most common clinically encountered patterns of orgasmic situations and some impressions about them:

I. *Lifelong absence of orgasmic experience*—this is what is usually thought of when the diagnosis of anorgasmia is made. This pattern suggests a limited comfort with intense sexual expression.

   A. *Adequate desire and arousal*—the problem seems to be the inability to get beyond the plateau level of arousal. This is the point at which orgasmic women begin to unself-consciously move their pelvises against the partner in order to trigger-off orgasm.

B. *Limited desire and arousal experience*—often desire problems in disguise. The anorgasmia is usually better considered in terms of the difficulty with drive, motive, and basic arousal.

II. *Lifelong absence of orgasm with partners*—this pattern suggests a limited trust of the safety and wisdom of sharing the sexual self with a partner. The clinician should be highly interested in what types of experiences the woman has had that have left her untrusting. These may have been sexual or nonsexual in nature and may involve each of the time periods of childhood, adolescence, and adulthood.

A. *Easy current attainment of orgasm with masturbation*—focus should eventually include the fantasies that accompany masturbation because they often provide hints as to the nature of the woman's traumatic experiences that lay behind her inability to trust.
   1. With a particular fantasy theme—sometimes the fantasies are only minor variations of the same visual story. The story is important to the woman even when it is seemingly a conventional romantic tale.
   2. Without a particular fantasy theme—fantasies are the imaginal keys, the conditions, for unlocking the woman's arousal mechanisms. The fantasies may derive from the woman's earlier experiences or borrowed from media exposure. When the woman uses a variety of fantasies, the clinician should attempt to perceive a common theme. Failing to do so, the therapist might try to consider with the woman what elements of the fantasy seem to be the most exciting. This can then be related to her current life circumstances.

B. *Past but not current attainment of orgasm with masturbation*—clinicians should be interested in when and why the masturbation ceased. Sometimes it is the occurrence of a frightening fantasy or the emergence of a painful memory that causes the woman to abandon the use of her body for her own pleasure.
   1. With a particular past fantasy theme
   2. No particular past fantasy theme

III. *Loss of orgasmic attainment with partner*—may be due to interpersonal, personal, or organic factors. The clinician needs to understand what was occurring in the woman's life when orgasmic attainment was lost. Masturbation pattern may be of no help because many women have not masturbated in years or are unable to honestly share this information with the clinician.

A. *Loss of orgasmic attainment with masturbation*—drug-induced anorgasmia, for example, with fluoxetane, often makes the masturbatory orgasm extremely difficult or impossible to attain.

B. *Preservation of orgasmic attainment with masturbation*—suggests more psychological or relationship factors are playing a role.

IV. *Easily orgasmic with one method but not during intercourse*—this is the most commonly encountered orgasmic situation among patients. Women are orgasmic, but not during intercourse. Their orgasmic attainment may be easy, regular, and psychologically satisfying, yet they or their partner may be concerned about the absence of orgasm during intercourse.

A. *Hand stimulation of the genitals*—this common form of orgasmic attainment may be the only method because of the woman's sensibilities about mouth stimulation of her genitals. With the authoritative mentioning of oral stimulation, some couples add this other means of orgasmic stimulation to their repertoire.

B. *Mouth stimulation of the genitals*—some woman experience the telling about their orgasms during oral stimulation to be an invasion of privacy and will not initially acknowledge that they are orgasmic in this way.

C. *Vibrator stimulation of the genitals*—women who are orgasmic only with a vibrator seem more sexually inhibited than those who can easily have orgasms with manual or oral stimulation. The vibrator seems to provide a mechanical override mechanism to psychological inhibition for some women. The vibrator does not induce orgasms in every woman.

V. *Difficult and unpredictable orgasmic attainment with partner*—many anorgasmic women attain orgasms on occasion. Sometimes, even though they have been orgasmic, they have had to work much too hard for too long to attain it. Sometimes, they are orgasmic in an exceptionally uninhibited experience by virtue of romantic setting, alcohol, or exposure to sexually explicit media. But their typical pattern is anorgasmia as in number I in this outline.

A. *Orgasmic with a particular fantasy*—the clinician remains interested in the fantasy that may accompany orgasm under these exceptional circumstances because it sometimes contains a clue to the nature of the woman's underlying inhibiting life experiences.

B. *Fantasy has no relationship to orgasmic attainment.*

USEFUL IDEAS FOR ANORGASMIC WOMEN

Here are some succinctly stated ideas that clinicians may find helpful for their anorgasmic patients. They are a mixture of fact, encouragement, and behavioral suggestions. Each of them may emotionally jar some patients because they have long behaved as though quite the opposite was true.

Ideas alone do not cure most people who come to a therapist. The therapist tactfully presents ideas in a manner that is designed for the individual person. These ideas provoke feelings and associations and come to be understood by the patient and the therapist as having a personal meaning to them. To the extent that these ideas are the missing cognitive pieces of information in the mental life of anorgasmic women, the therapy invariably touches on most of these notions. Clinicians are not likely to confuse reading such a list with the processes of digesting, assimilating, or working through these ideas in therapy, even though some women may have sufficient readiness to hear or read these ideas that they become orgasmic without discussion with anyone else.

1. You are not biologically defective.
2. Orgasmic attainment is possible.
3. You are responsible for your orgasmic attainment.
4. Orgasm will not be brought to you through passive behavior under most sexual circumstances.
5. The clitoris is your sexual organ.
6. You can learn how to move your pelvis in various ways to stimulate your clitoris.
7. Your partner can only help so much, the rest must be done actively by you.
8. Orgasm is the result of progressively focusing attention on pelvic sensations.
9. Intense pelvic sensations are normal, legitimate, and healthy.
10. A several-minute, single-minded concentration on the self is required to create an orgasm during intercourse or direct clitoral stimulation.
11. The concentration of your sensations is not selfishness; it is your way of claiming the sensual aspects of yourself. It will simultaneously provide pleasure to you and your partner.
12. Orgasm requires muscular work.
13. There are very good reasons why you are not allowing yourself to be more sexually excited. Therapy is the process by which you and I define and understand these reasons.

THE DEEPER MEANINGS OF ORGASMIC INHIBITION

After a short while with a therapist, it becomes clear to a woman that she is the one who is limiting her arousal. She is the one who is running away from the sexual scene when there is a possibility of becoming more aroused. This mystery, having been solved, is quickly replaced by another: Why am I doing this?

In the case history that we examined earlier, Kate had several reasons: she was afraid of all emotional intensity and she wanted to be a good girl. Women inhibit themselves for their own reasons. The elucidation of the specific reasons in a woman's life is one of the pleasures of therapy. The individuality of the reasons of each anorgasmic woman keeps the therapy interesting for the clinician.

There are two important commonly occurring ideas that are found among anorgasmic women. The first one is that the woman ends her participation in lovemaking because the emotion of sexual arousal is linked in her mind to problematic past excitements. One woman told me, "I used to lie on my father's bed with him and snuggle. He often was so tired and depressed and I would comfort and stroke him until he fell asleep. When I was making love for the first time with Ray, I thought of my father and got scared. Suddenly, it was like I was having sex with my father." The orgasm that is not attained is a symbol of something forbidden. The woman wants to repress, suppress, or otherwise avoid painful memories. The painful memories may involve actual sexual abuse, sexually exciting relationships with a father that do not include inappropriate touching, or longings for closeness with a parent who was distant, destructive, or highly problematic. Many of these matters used to be summarized as Oedipal problems.

The second important idea for clinicians is that although orgasmic attainment problems do not have a consistent underlying cause, anorgasmia is a form of defense that is protecting the woman from something that is anxiety provoking. Once this is appreciated by the patient and the therapist, the task of therapy switches from attaining orgasms to finding out what painful memory, affects, or conflicts are being defended against with the symptom. If the clinician can help the woman deal with and work through this pain, she will be in a far better position to use the helpful ideas and behavioral suggestions. If, however, the clinician just prescribes masturbation exercises or explains how the female-on-top position and "bumping and grinding" of her pelvis can augment her sensations, the woman is not likely to be helped because she still has the need to avoid the mental processes of her own excitement. The woman has a sexual learning problem because it is worth it to her to be sexually dysfunctional rather than to recall her past experiences. Once this is clear between the two of them, therapy may efficiently proceed. Both the therapist and the patient have to have respect for the resistance.

SUMMARY

Women are correct when they expect to attain orgasm during partner sexual experiences. Orgasmic attainment is usually so highly valued by women and their partners that when orgasms do not regularly occur, negative feelings and erroneous accusations often adversely affect the sexual equilibrium. Therapists can be helpful to some of these women. The clinical process begins with a careful history, including questions about masturbation, in order to determine the situations in which orgasms have been experienced. This enables a discrimination between personal intolerance of intense arousal, an inability to feel safe with any partner, isolation from the culture's recent encouragement of women's sexual expression, a deteriorated nonsexual relationship, organic factors, and simple difficulties coordinating arousing behaviors with the partner. Although a number of succinct ideas are often helpful to women with orgasmic inhibition, some women need to work through the deeper personal meanings of their symptom before these ideas will be useful. This requires individual psychotherapy for many women.

REFERENCES

1. Waterman CK, Chiavzzi EJ: The role of orgasm in male and female sexual enjoyment. *Journal of Sex Research* 18:146–159, 1982.
2. McCabe MP, Delaney SM: An evaluation of therapeutic programs for the treatment of secondary inorgasmia in women. *Archives of Sexual Behavior*, 1992; 21(1):69–89.
3. Masters WH, Johnson V: *Human Sexual Inadequacy.* Boston, Little, Brown, 1970.
4. Masters WH, Johnson V: *Human Sexual Response.* Boston, Little, Brown, 1966.
5. LoPiccolo J, Lobitz WC: The role of masturbation in the treatment of orgasmic inhibition. *Archives of Sexual Behavior*, 1972; 2:163–171.
6. Barbach L: *For Yourself: A Guide to Female Sexual Fulfillment.* New York, Doubleday, 1982.
7. Barbach L: Group treatment of anorgasmic women, in Lieblum SR, Pervin LA (eds), *Principles and Practices of Sex Therapy.* New York, Guilford, 1980.
8. Kurianski JB, Sharpe L, O'Connor D: The treatment of anorgasmia: Long-term effectiveness of a short-term behavioral group therapy. *Journal of Sex and Marital Therapy*, 1982; 8:29–43.
9. Libman E, Fichten CS, Brender W, *et al.*: A comparison of three therapeutic formats in the treatment of secondary orgasmic dysfunction. *Journal of Sex and Marital Therapy*, 1984; 10:147–159.
10. Killman PR, Mills KH, Caid C, *et al.*: Treatment of secondary orgasmic dysfunction: An outcome study. *Archives of Sexual Behavior*, 1986; 15:211–229.

CHAPTER 10

Erection Problems

The penis is attached to the heart. It is the male organ of emotional connection. The psycho-genically impotent man's penis knows something that his conscious mind is not permitted to realize; it should be trusted.

Impotence, as erectile problems have traditionally been known, brings the mental health professional into the province of the medical doctor[1]. The clinical work with these high-prevalence problems requires knowledge of the mechanisms of erection, physical disease processes, the impact of medications, the value of diagnostic tests, the utility of mechanical interventions, and the limitations of the clinical method. Psychotherapists should not run from this challenge. The correct diagnosis and therapy often require input from one professional who expertly perceives organic pathophysiology and one who has a profound grasp of the psychology of the problem. Few physicians know both subjects well enough to adequately treat most impotent men alone.

FOUR GENERIC TYPES OF ERECTILE DYSFUNCTION

The diagnostic evaluation of impotence begins with a man's complaint of an inability to have intercourse because of a soft or absent erection when he believes a firm, lasting erection is reasonable. At its conclusion, his problem is placed into one of four categories—psychogenic, organic, mixed, or idiopathic, and then is further delineated in terms of specific etiologic factors. This is accomplished by integrating three groups of data: the pattern of the erections; the social and psychological events preceding the onset of the symptom; and the physical examination and laboratory findings. When the etiologic factors are individually appreciated, treatment options can be considered. The four steps of the clinical process—

evaluation, diagnostic grouping, etiologic specification, and treatment—should not taken out of order.

THE DIAGNOSIS OF PSYCHOGENIC IMPOTENCE

Erectile Pattern

The patient is placed in the psychogenic category when the clinician recognizes that the man's neural, vascular, and endocrine capacities to generate adequate erections are intact. *Selective erectile dysfunction* is the diagnostic hallmark of psychogenic impotence: Despite the fact that the man cannot initiate or maintain reliable erections with a partner, he consistently does so under other circumstances.

The presence of a stand-up, rigid, lasting erection when intercourse is not being attempted usually alerts the clinician to psychogenic impotence. These adequate erections occur during the night or early morning, during kissing or petting behaviors, during masturbation, with certain partners, in response to magazines or videos, or spontaneously. The clinician looks for an inconstant physical factor, such as intermittent substance abuse or medication use, that might explain the selective pattern. Lacking this, the diagnosis of psychogenic impotence seems to jump out at the clinician, at least in young men.

The diagnosis is easiest to make in young men because their drive, ease of arousal, and degree of responsiveness to erotic stimuli are great. The recognition of psychogenic impotence from the pattern of erections becomes more difficult during midlife because sexual neurophysiology slows. Erections are more easily suppressed in midlife by the affect states that accompany marital problems, vocational disappointments, and concerns over children.

Since research has demonstrated that the frequency, duration, and fullness of nocturnal erections are significantly impaired by depression,[2] the clinician must be careful not to use erection patterns alone when making this diagnosis in a middle-aged man who is experiencing social and psychological misery. The clinician needs to weigh judiciously the infrequently adequate erection against the man's emotional state.

The consideration of the man's emotional circumstances is even more important in men over 55 because psychogenic impotence may be present despite the fact that no adequate erections have been detected by the man for many months. If much has changed in the man's life before the onset of the erectile problem, psychogenic impotence should not be quickly ruled out. In this age group, misdiagnosis is often made because not enough significance is given to the social history.

The Social and Psychological History

Psychogenic erectile dysfunction is usefully classified as primary and secondary. *Primary impotence* is that which has been present throughout life—the man has never been able to have intercourse. The far more prevalent cases of *secondary impotence* occur after a long period of successful intercourse. The social and psychological changes that typically precede secondary impotence involve: relationship alienation; divorce; death of a spouse; vocational failure; and loss of personal or spousal health. Each of these circumstances triggers impotence by eliciting feelings and conflicts that interfere with potency.

The social and the psychological histories among those with primary impotence are quite different. Since potency has never been securely present, the history usually spontaneously focuses on childhood and adolescent developmental matters. The topics of sexual identity, general personality functioning, and psychiatric diagnostic issues quickly become foremost in the clinician's mind.

The Specific Psychological Disorder

The evaluation allows the therapist to extend the diagnosis beyond psychogenic impotence to hypothesize the type of issue that the patient is struggling with—widower's impotence, marital discord, homosexuality, depression. These will be considered further later in this chapter.

The Laboratory Findings

The laboratory can be helpful in recognizing psychogenic impotence when the pattern of erections is ambiguous, the antecedent events are not striking, and the patient and the therapist need to know the etiology within a short time period. Generally speaking the laboratory tests are entirely normal. The prototype test is the overnight measurement of penile tumescence and rigidity in a laboratory.[3]

The patient sleeps in a special room equipped to monitor his brain waves, extraocular muscles, neck muscles, oxygen saturation, and penile activity. Two nights are usually sufficient. Nondepressed men with psychogenic impotence resemble aged-matched normal men in the sleep laboratory. They have at least three episodes of tumescence (more for younger men) lasting from 10 to 30 minutes each throughout the night. These episodes usually occur every 60 to 90 minutes and coincide with rapid eye movements and dreaming.

The penile tumescence is measured by attaching a looped mercury strain around the base and end of the shaft of the penis. Rigidity is measured by waking the patient and asking him about his erection's strength and measuring its buckling pressure. While many men have trouble sleeping the first night and do not obtain conclusive results, others can have a one-night-only test because it is clear that they have normal erections. The sleep laboratory is expensive, time consuming, disruptive of patient's normal routines, and requires considerable technological expertise. Under the best of hands, this test can be expected to provide an accurate assessment in approximately 80% of cases. Considering the problems of false negatives, false positives, and the confounding impact of depression and age, this is a highly respectable figure.

Some clinics that specialize in erectile problems use a take-home device called a *RigiScan* as a substitute for sleep laboratory assessment.[4] The RigiScan provides two strain gauges to measure tumescence and rigidity at the base and the top of the penis. It does not measure sleep parameters. The norms for the RigiScan are not as well developed as for the sleep laboratory. Nonetheless, the RigiScan and similar devices are in use because of lower cost and convenience.

Individual physicians sometimes provide the patient with simpler devices to measure their nocturnal events. These include the *Snap-Gauge*, which is a relatively inexpensive band containing three ribbons of differing tensile strengths that is placed around the penis.[5] When all ribbons are broken, the patient is presumed to have had strong nocturnal erections. An even simpler device is a roll of vertically perforated stamps which are pasted on the penile shaft. If the perforations are split by morning, the man is presumed to have had strong nocturnal erections. Neither the RigiScan nor the simpler devices have been thoroughly assessed for *sensitivity* (percentage of organic cases that are missed—false negatives) and *specificity* (percentage of psychogenic cases that are diagnosed as organic—false positives) and, therefore, do not provide the same degree of diagnostic confidence that a well-run sleep laboratory does.

THE DIAGNOSIS OF ORGANIC IMPOTENCE

Erectile Pattern

The suspicion of organic impotence is raised by a history of a consistent upper level of erection deficit. Erectile variations in the degree of enlargement, capacity to be upright, duration, and rigidity are common in organic cases. The best erections tend to occur upon awakening. Erections tend to decrease in adequacy in this order; middle of the night or morning; masturbation; foreplay; and intercourse. Despite the variation, an erectile deficit is apparent. The penis may never be full, rigid, erect, or last more than a brief time.

It often is useful to ask the man to numerically rate his erections. For instance, if a full, lasting, stand-up erection is designated 10, a typical organic pattern may look like this: mornings—6; masturbation—4 to 6; foreplay—3 to 4; intercourse—0 to 3. The variations probably reflect the influence of anxiety about obtaining and maintaining the erection. This type of anxiety is called *performance anxiety.* It is routinely noticed among impotent men in all diagnostic categories. Performance anxiety is the vigilant preoccupation with the state of erection that keeps the man from sensually experiencing lovemaking. Rather than giving himself over to the pleasures of touching and being touched, he thinks about how adequate his erection is or will be.

The anticipation and dread of the loss of erection is highly destructive; it precludes arousal by substituting anxiety and inattention to sensation. In men with organic impotence, this almost inescapable mental process adds another deficit to the one brought about by the erection-impairing disease. Performance anxiety causes men to go through the motions of lovemaking, instead of participating in a relaxed sensual manner.

There is a mystery about the organic erectile pattern that merits emphasis. Many men with organic deficit patterns for long periods of time occasionally have a good morning erection. This history leaves the clinician wondering. Does the man really have psychogenic impotence? Is the neural pathway for the noctural erection physiologically distinct from that which mediates waking erections? Are psychological and organic influences a part of every case of impotence? Is it possible for organically impaired erectile mechanisms to be overridden by sufficient nocturnal psychic stimulation?

The variations in the pattern of erections found among the organically impaired are further explained by four medical facts. Organic impotence is caused by a large number of diseases whose pathophysiologies are distinct from one another—for example, multiple sclerosis subverts erections in the spinal cord by blocking neurotransmission, whereas antihypertensive agents interfere with brain and peripheral neural mechanisms. The same impotence-producing diseases vary in severity from patient to patient—for example, atherosclerosis can cause erections to hover between 0 and 2 if there are extensive blockages of aortoiliac-hypogastric arterial flow or it can account for erections of 7 or 8 if only one more distal artery is blocked. In addition, one disease may impair potency through multiple mechanisms. Diabetes, for instance, may lead to the loss of nerve fibers in the penis, the loss of neurotransmitter mechanisms for vasodilation of the sinusoids, and a decrement of desire and arousal from poor metabolic control and renal disease.

The Specific Organic Diagnoses

Easy-to-diagnose organic impotence is associated with an illness that is known to cause erectile dysfunction. For instance, either the patient already has diabetes, severe atherosclerosis, multiple sclerosis, severe hypertension, carcinoma of the prostate, ulcerative colitis that has been treated with a colectomy, or is newly diagnosed by a physician to have an organic factor, such as congestive heart failure, pituitary tumor, severe anemia, alcoholic cirrhosis, or Peyronie's disease. An organic erectile pattern without a specified causal disease or medication is a reason for caution. Is this psychogenic impotence? Is there a subtle hormonal, neural, or systemic disease that is being missed?

I. Vascular
  A. Atherosclerosis of arteries providing blood to cavernous spaces—iliac-hypogastric-pudendal-penile-cavernosal system
  B. Arteriosclerosis of penile, cavernosal, and helicine arteries
  C. Sinusoidal dysfunction
  D. Venous leakage
  E. Blunt or irradiation trauma to arteries supplying the cavernous spaces
  F. Intrapenile vascular damage from priapism

II. Neural
  A. Brain deficits
  B. Spinal cord deficits
  C. Ganglia and peripheral nerve deficits
  D. Intrapenile nerve deficits

III. Endocrine
  A. Hypogonadism from hyper- and hypogonadotrophic conditions
  B. Prolactin excess from pituitary tumor, medication use, renal failure
  C. Panhypopituitarism
  D. Hypo- and hyperthyroidism

IV. Systemic illnesses
  A. Cardio-respiratory failure
  B. Renal failure
  C. Retroperitoneal tumors

V. Medications
  A. Antihypertensive agents
  B. Hypogonadal agents
  C. Chronic use of anticonvulsants
  D. High doses of phenothiazines and antidepressants
  E. Antineoplastic agents

VI. Surgery
  A. Removal of prostatic capsule
  B. Involving the retroperitoneal space such as for

1. Repair of aortic aneurysm
2. Lymph node dissections
3. Sigmoid colon and rectum removal

VII. Pelvic radiation

Social History

In easy-to-diagnose organic impotence, nothing dramatic has changed prior to or along with the decrements in erectile functioning. A wife's affair, a job loss, a child's drug abuse, an unhappy relationship affair, depression—the types of histories that are often obtained from men with secondary psychogenic impotence are *not* obtained in men with easy-to-diagnose organic illness. The patient and his partner testify that life is fine but his erections are not.

The Laboratory

Sleep laboratory findings only suggest an organic pattern; they do not localize the problem. In addition to the blood studies that are a routine part of a medical evaluation, the complaint of impotence directs the physician to order the serum testosterone level and, if it is low a second time, to order pituitary and other hormone levels.

Urologists use special laboratory studies to examine the arterial, sinusoidal, and venous capacities of the penis. The simplest of these is the measurement of blood pressure in the flaccid penis. A pediatric cuff is inflated on the distal shaft and the first systolic pulse is listened for with a Doppler stethoscope. The systolic blood pressure measured on the arm is then used to calculate the penile-brachial index (PBI) by dividing the penile pressure by the brachial pressure. PBIs over 0.8 are thought to be normal; under 0.7 indicative of arterial blockage; and between 0.7 and 0.8 indeterminant. Because the specificity and sensitivity of the PBI are not impressive, diagnoses of arteriogenic impotence are not based on PBI findings alone.

Other tests aim to evaluate the penis in the erect state[6]: the Duplex ultrasonographic visualizations of the cavernosal arteries; measuring intracavernosal pressures; papaverine injections; use of radiopaque dyes. None of these tests has been standardized on potent age-matched controls. All have uncertain sensitivities and specificities. Individual urologists, however, may place considerable importance on their findings because they refine the organic explanations to penile arteriosclerosis, sinusoidal dysfunction, or venous leakage using physiologic data.

THE DIAGNOSIS OF MIXED IMPOTENCE

The category of mixed impotence is used when a man with an organic cause, such as diabetic or alcoholic peripheral neuropathy or antihypertensive medication, has an additional significant contribution from his social or psychological life. A medicated, hypertensive, diabetic whose wife is not talking to him, for instance, may be rendered impotent as a result of four factors: marital problems, depression, intrapenile nerve loss, and a calcium channel blocking agent. A 65-year-old man with supraventricular tachycardia who is taking 120 mg of propranolol may also be dealing with the implications of a myocardial infarction, an insecure job, and a child who has just been asked not to return to college. When men are judged to have mixed impotence, it is important to list the psychological and organic factors so that treatment planning can separately address each of them.

THE DIAGNOSIS OF IDIOPATHIC IMPOTENCE

When the clinician cannot identify the cause of a patient's erectile problem with reasonable certainty, the case is classified as *idiopathic*. Time often reveals the true diagnosis as organic or psychogenic—for example, a pelvic malignancy or marital deterioration is subsequently discovered. Some idiopathic impotence is simply an artifact of not including the partner in the evaluation process. Wives are well known for their ability to provide therapists with clarifying information about their husband's social and psychological state so that the correct diagnosis can be made. Even after thorough evaluations, however, there are cases in which the clinician does not know the cause of the erectile problem.

Recently, some progress has been made in clarifying some previously enigmatic cases. Masters and Johnson's observations that aging men find that their erections are slower to form, are not as rigid, and are shorter lasting have been rigorously scientifically confirmed. Using sleep laboratory, psychometric, and clinical evaluations of happily married, extremely physically healthy men, Schiavi and his co-workers documented a gradual decline in physiological capacities between 55 and 74 years of age.[7]

Two crucial ideas emerged from their careful work: the physiological mechanisms for the decline in erectile capacity with age are unknown since the decline was not related to the diseases that cause organic impotence; men with the same physiological decrements can be found among the impotent and the potent.

These observations direct clinicians to the psychosomatic basis of sexual functioning and to the sexual equilibrium. It is possible that some idiopathically impotent men may develop sufficient performance anxiety to undermine their potency in response to their own perception of erectile decline or their partner's comments about their erections. The partner may respond to the man's worries by avoiding lovemaking and quietly retiring from sex. She may do this to prevent his humiliation or because she is happy to stop having sex with him.

Idiopathic impotence is further generated by the decline in sexual drive that is usually apparent by the late fifties. Because the man is not as often and as intensely aroused spontaneously or in response to love-making, he can comfortably not make love for longer periods of time than earlier in his life. The decline in drive and the erectile decrements summate.

These nuances are difficult to perceive during the initial evaluation. Even after the couple is seen over an extended period of time, the situation may be missed. Clinicians need to guard against the mistake of assuming a case is organic when it is, in fact, idiopathic.

Nowhere in the adult life cycle is the term *impotence* more destructive to the man and his partner than among healthy men around 60 years of age. Many of these so-called impotent men are able to have intercourse. Their problem is that their erections are no longer predictable or reliable. Their problem is *erectile unreliability*—not impotence. This semantic shift means a great deal to these men and their partners. In this age group, impotence generally conveys that there is permanent loss of erectile capacity, whereas an unreliable penis implies that tomorrow may be a better day.

When idiopathic impotence occurs in a man younger than the early fifties, the clinician should worry about hidden organic and psychogenic factors. When it occurs during the late fifties and older, it is of great value to closely study the sexual equilibrium over time. There is likely to be a shifting balance of male and female arousability that sometimes makes intercourse possible and sometimes prevents it. Much idiopathic impotence may turn out to be mixed impotence because it combines a definite, though inconstant physiological decline with a subtle, fluctuating psychological factor, which at different times derives from performance anxiety and emotions about social changes.

A GENERAL SCHEME FOR THE PATHOGENESIS OF PSYCHOGENIC IMPOTENCE

Nonpsychiatric physicians treat psychogenic impotence as though it were one disease. Therapists do not have the luxury of this illusion; psychogenic impotence professionally belongs to psychotherapists. We know that it is merely a symptom of some underlying enigma. Although the enigmas are quite varied, they have a metaphor in common: Psychogenic impotence is a message that tells the man's body not to cooperate with intercourse. The symptom is almost always a partial mystery to the man because he cannot allow himself to understand how his social or psychological dilemmas affect his potency.

Contributions from Three Time Periods

Psychogenic impotence is usually generated by the resonating interaction of emotional forces from the present, the recent past, and childhood. Specifically, these are the performance anxieties that occur during lovemaking, the life events that precede the onset of the symptom, and developmental vulnerabilities from childhood and adolescent years.

Performance anxiety serves the man as a distraction from other feelings he may be having about making love in general and about making love to his particular partner. The psychogenically impotent man typically does not appreciate the significance of the life changes that preceded his impotence. He is either unsure of or denies the emotional meaning of these events. He fails to realize that his symptom is the result of these events and his responses to them. He focuses on his loss of sexual confidence (a frequent phrase for performance anxiety) as the cause of his problem; he remains befuddled about how he originally fell into its pernicious trap.

Part of the mystery of psychogenic impotence derives from events of long ago. Intercourse or intercourse with his partner acquires meanings that derive from experiences much earlier in life. Therapists tend to describe these meanings in varying ways: failed tasks of psychological development, impairments in sexual identity, vulnerabilities of the self-system, Oedipal issues, various forms of abuse, social learning difficulties, pregenital fixations, and transference.

The resonation of forces from these three spheres of time provides a scheme for understanding both secondary and primary psychogenic impotence. A scheme is only a skeletal outline of the process of symptom generation and maintenance. The clinician works to add the flesh during the evaluation and the therapy by noting the extent of performance anxiety, pinpointing the precipitating events, and defining their emotional meanings.

THE PRECIPITANTS OF SECONDARY PSYCHOGENIC IMPOTENCE

Secondary psychogenic impotence occurs under diverse social and psychological circumstances. It is triggered by the destructive impact of feelings that successfully compete for arousal during sex play. These feelings typically stem from one of the five social changes described below. The newly impotent man does not recognize the emotional significance of this change or its relationship to his potency. The affects associated with the impotence-triggering event soon are amplified by their similarities to past developmental experiences. For some people, making love seems to create a confrontation with one's own psychic truths. Performance anxiety, which usually begins after one or two erectile failures, helps the man to avoid thinking about these truths. Men are vulnerable to the development of this symptom to the degree to which they are characterized by the expectation that they ought to be able to perform sexually regardless of social circumstances and by the inability to quickly experience and understand their affects.

Relationship Deterioration

The self-declaration of impotence in the face of alienation, mutual hostility, lack of psychological intimacy, and partner unreceptivity is a testimony to the man's expectation that he and his penis ought to be able to function under any conditions. Such optimism is not warranted even though the shocked man may emphasize that, in his last marriage, he was able to have intercourse when divorcing. It is reasonable for the clinician to presume that such a man's impotence involves some of the following: resentment; loneliness; confusion about who is correct about the couple's unresolved differences; guilt over his role in their troubles; reaction to his partner's unreceptivity and anger; fear of abandonment; and helplessness to end their downward spiral.

> A 37-year-old successful lawyer became impotent with his wife, had his first extramarital affair, and was impotent with his lover for two months. Once he recovered his potency, he divorced his wife and married his lover. "I didn't realize how angry I was at my wife, but I did know how guilty and unsure I was with my lover at first. I was angry at my wife because nothing I did was good enough; everything was a hassle with her, including my having to beg for sex." When asked to state the single most powerful reason for his anger at her, he quickly replied, "She stopped liking me! Without that, I could not function."

Divorce

Many divorcing and divorced men are surprised by their embarrassing sexual difficulty. Initially, they cannot relate their bitterness, guilt, or fear of future attachment to their erection problem. They, too, expect their penises to operate autonomously. It is reasonable for the clinician to presume that such a man's impotence involves some of the following: love for his wife; fear of his rage at women; doubt about his lovability; doubt about his ability to love; despair over his children's pain and alienation; wariness that the new partner will eventually turn into an impossible person as his wife did; and guilt over his dishonesty with new partners.

A gentle, highly principled man who did not want a divorce slowly came to perceive that he was the victim of his cruel materialistic wife, who by cunning and guile took his assets and turned his two young sons against him. Although he felt he knew the real reason for his wife's requests for extra funds and frequent family crises that required her to be away, he always quietly acceded to her requests. His lawyer told him that he was crazy for not taking steps to preserve his wealth. However, he was doing what he felt was correct to maximize his attachments to his sons and to give his wife a chance for a happier life. When he eventually began dating, he was impotent. While he acknowledged only sadness about his wife's behavior, he had nightmares about violence and terror. He eventually learned to feel his rage in therapy but, in doing so, he first experienced his fear of its expression and could appreciate how it threatened his self-concept as a kind, gentle, peace-loving person.

Death of Spouse

Most widowers are at least in their fifties. Their feelings about resuming a sexual life with a new partner are influenced by many factors, such as the duration and quality of the marriage, the cause of their wives' deaths, and their own health. Many of these men have been through slow deaths from cancer, and began mourning well before the actual event. Because there are many partners available to physically healthy widowers, many men use dating as a distraction from being home alone and other inevitably difficult aspects of grief. It is reasonable for the clinician to presume that the impotence of recent widowers involves some of the following: unresolved grief; guilt about impulses to have multiple partners; sense that he belongs only to his wife; confusion about his new freedom; discomfort about his children's and friends' reactions of his dating and the specific women he dates.

Breast cancer began when his wife was 47, and took her life four surgeries, two chemotherapy courses, and 7 years later. Their sexual life persisted for 6 years ending eventually because of her weakness. Three months after her death, he had his first date. It was with a woman who he quickly recognized was not a candidate as his next wife. Sex was aproblematic. Three months later, he had one date with a lovely woman who had had a mastectomy; he felt that he could not "go through it again" and never called her back. When he found a woman he thought he might eventually be able to marry, he was impotent for the first time in his life.

Vocational Failure

Vocational adequacy is central to most men's identity and self-esteem. Vocational failure or threatened vocational failure creates feelings of despair, uncertainty, anxiety, unworthiness, and guilt, which may be most apparent when the man attempts to make love. "I don't feel worthy of her any longer," may lurk behind the recent impotence of men with employment problems.

> One year prior to retirement, a usually prudent businessman made a bad investment and lost 25% of the money he and his wife were to live on during retirement. The remaining funds were adequate for their life-style, but "the added luxuries were probably not going to be possible." His wife was not nearly as disturbed by this loss as he was. Neither recognized that his new impotence was related to this business problem because he had weathered financial difficulties in the past without sexual symptoms. This man blamed himself for foolishly trusting a man who promised him too much. He felt that he was not worthy of his loving wife, who was loyal, proud, and ever-respectful of him.

Loss of Personal or Spousal Health

Psychogenic potency problems are common after major health events, such as myocardial infarction, open heart surgery, stroke, or cancer. Fear of death during sexual activity or a heightened awareness of the recent close call may be most apparent to the man during lovemaking. The partner's reactions to the man's illness and new health status may not be completely worked through, and can create a subtle sexual unreceptivity that triggers erectile failure and performance anxiety. This is a two-way system: the deterioration of the partner's health may also lead to erectile impairment because of his new perceptions of his partner.

> A retired man whose major occupation had become caring for his wife, who had Alzheimer's disease, became impotent during the second year of her care. Their sexual life continued, despite her increasing difficulties, fueled by their new closeness, the loss of her previous pattern of delaying responding to his request for sex, and the fact that she seemed to enjoy it. As she developed incontinence and began aimless nocturnal wanderings, he began having erectile failures. He simultaneously understood and was mystified by his impotence. "It just was not right any more; she was too sick."

> A happily married man was supportive when his younger second wife had a mastectomy. When she came home and wanted to have sex, he was eager and potent. Within several days, however, she began insisting that he look at her chest wall. He knew that it was not a wise thing for him to do because he had always been squeamish about blood and bodily injury. He begged for more time, but she insisted that she needed him to see the new her and to deal with her "half-chest" as she must. He looked and thereafter could not make love. She was furious; he was guilty. A long intense period of marital distress ensued.

PRIMARY PSYCHOGENIC IMPOTENCE

Primary psychogenic impotence may be defined stringently or liberally. The stringent definition includes only those men who have absolutely never been able to have vaginal intercourse. The liberal definition includes men who occasionally have been able to have intercourse, but who usually cannot. A guess of the relative prevalence in the general population of men at age 30 is 0.5% for the stringent cases versus 5.0% for the liberal ones.

Immediate antecedent life events do not seem to play a major role in the pathogenesis of stringently defined primary impotence. While performance anxiety is usually very much in evidence, the key elements of pathogenesis derive from remote developmental processes that leave the male intensely frightened of, or genuinely disinterested in, intercourse. Immediate antecedent life events seem to play a minor role among the liberally defined cases.

The causes of primary psychogenic impotence are related to those factors that explain the man's private sense of himself as inadequate and his strong, inarticulate fears of closeness to a woman. These powerful issues generate an emotional state that either precludes arousal entirely or overwhelms the physiological impact of arousal.

Among some men with primary impotence, intercourse is possible when certain unusual conditions of fantasy or behavior are met. These conditions typically involve meeting unconventional sexual identity needs, such as being partially dressed in women's attire or fantasizing being with a man. When conducting an evaluation of a man with primary impotence, careful consideration should be given to each of the three components of sexual identity. Clinicians should not be surprised when, after initial denials, the patient reveals an unconventional eroticism involving gender identity, orientation, or intention.

Some men with primary impotence come to clinical attention because of the lack of sexual desire. Most of these men have adequate sexual drive with a strong motivation to avoid sexual behavior with a partner.

Unlike secondary impotence in which there is no necessary relationship between a DSM-III-R diagnosis and the sexual dysfunction, primary impotence is often, though not invariably, associated with a diagnosable major condition. Most of these conditions are Axis II diagnoses, such as obsessive-compulsive, schizoid, or borderline personality; some, however, have a significant Axis I problem, such as depression, psychosis, or anxiety disorder.

Gender Identity Problems

This is the least common of the sexual identity difficulties that lurk behind primary impotence. Most of these men are considered transvestites. They acknowledge having recurrent fantasies of being a woman, of cross-dressing in private, of discovering that their potency is assured by wearing a female garment during lovemaking, or by thinking that their partner's breasts and vagina are their own.

> An impotent man who had been married for 3 months confessed to his sturdy, alcohol-dependent, determined-to-get-to-the-bottom-of-this wife that he had been cross-dressing since age 14. Much to his surprise, she asked to see him dressed. They talked a great deal, became closer than ever. When he asked if he could make love wearing "his" slip, they were able to consummate their relationship. Her tolerance for his cross-dressing waxed and waned; when he could not wear "something," his potency was impaired or marginal as was his desire for lovemaking.

Homoeroticism

The most common source of primary impotence in many settings is homoeroticism. Many men who have responded with arousal to male bodies and repeatedly masturbated to male images cannot calmly make the transition from their homoeroticism to a homosexual identity and life-style. Some of them attempt a heterosexual relationship and fail at intercourse, seemingly because the motivational aspects of their sexual desire are lacking. They may never have revealed their homoeroticism to their partners and often will not spontaneously reveal it to the clinician. Their performance anxiety seems to grow when they cannot sustain arousal during lovemaking.

> A highly successful corporate executive, active in Alcoholics Anonymous for 15 years since attaining sobriety, masturbates to homoerotic images when he is away on his frequent business trips, but has never had sexual contact with a man. Although he has had intercourse with his wife during their 18 years of marriage, the frequency has been once or twice a year during the last decade. In the early years of marriage, the highest frequency of attempts was monthly, and he was impotent about half the time. When potent, he felt he needed to get it over with as quickly as possible. He typically responds with silence to his wife's entreaties for an explanation, or simply says, "I don't know why, but I can't." He resisted her requests for professional help until he thought she was going to abandon him. The first therapist failed to ask about his eroticism and the patient never volunteered the information.

Paraphilia

Men with longstanding, highly arousing, unusual erotic fantasies that are associated with a compulsion to masturbate or act out with a partner usually have some impairment of conventional heterosexual function as well.[8] This impairment is most often manifested as an avoidance of lovemaking, but it also commonly involves impotence or inability to ejaculate in the vagina. The presence of the paraphilia usually must be directly elicited from the patient by careful questioning.

> Before the AIDS epidemic, a sheepish high school teacher in his late fifties asked to be put in contact with a sex surrogate because he wanted to be able to have intercourse once before he died. Although he dated occasionally for social reasons, he had never had any physical intimacy with anyone but a prostitute. His eroticism was dominated by the image of being spanked. He masturbated several times a day to variations on this theme, and had arranged elaborate means of hurting himself during masturbation. All attempts at intercourse with prostitutes had failed; during the last decade, he had only requested to be yelled at and spanked for his naughtiness.

Abuse History

Heterosexual potency requires two capacities: to be aroused by a woman and to be able to neutralize the ordinary fear and nervousness about entering her body. Sexual identity problems limit the capacity to respond to women with arousal. When those with serious sexual identity problems are excluded, however, a large group of men who cannot neutralize their anxiety about lovemaking remain. These young men transfer feelings toward their parents or other earlier significant attachments to partner because of the unconscious assumption that she will hurt him just as "they" did. The hurt may have been the result of egregious psychological abandonment, beatings, sexual abuse, and prolonged overly close relationships with their mothers. The patient's problem indicates that he is pessimistic about finding anyone who is trustworthy enough to share his bodily experience with him.

> A 22-year-old sought help because of his consistent inability to erect with women. He feared that he would never be able to marry, love, and have a family because he was not aroused by the women that attracted him. "Nothing arouses me anymore!" The problem seemed to stem from the periodic sexual abuse he experienced from his 5-year-older cousin during his 9th and 10th years of life. The teenager often tied him up, fondled his genitals, and forced him to do the same to him. He threatened violence but also told him that there was nothing wrong with what they were doing. "All boys do this." This did not prevent the patient's shame and subsequent fear of being excited lest he recall the excitements and humiliations of his youth.

> A passive-dependent man, who has never enjoyed a reliable potency during his 25 years of marriage, was the only child of a woman who was widowed at age 27, when he was 30 months old. Although she dated briefly when he was 8, he was the sole male in her life until he married. His wife complained that she had to do everything for him, like a mother. He refused to make any decisions, wanted to be waited on hand and foot, and seemed

lost outside of his work environment, where, if he strayed too far from his wife, he was susceptible to panicky feelings.

PSYCHOTHERAPY

To the patient, the diagnosis of psychogenic impotence initially means that the problem is not physical. To the therapist, the symptom usually means that the man does not feel safe in emotionally attaching to another person. The therapist is safe in assuming that the symptom is the patient's way of resolving a hidden drama between his wishes for sexual intercourse and his fears about the consequences of emotional attachment. Therapy needs to provide the patient with dignity, understanding, the opportunity to feel, and the chance to become better acquainted with how his mind operates. Therapy gives the man a chance to find a less burdensome, more direct manner of expressing his private feelings about himself and his situation.

One of the clinician's early therapy choices is whether to see the man alone or with his partner. Partners usually need attention because, being part of the sexual equilibrium, they either play a role in the genesis of the symptom or are strongly affected by it. Conjoint therapy can be efficient and effective for impotence that is heavily derived from recent interpersonal conflicts in faithful couples. Conjoint therapy can prevent symptom resolution, however, when the man needs to discuss his sexual identity, his inadequate sense of self, his persistent desires for other partners, or his childhood experiences that have left him deceitful, distrusting, and wary of closeness. Conjoint therapy is also not wise when the clinician has reason to believe that honesty will not be possible. Currently or recently unfaithful husbands should not be seen in conjoint therapies unless the infidelity is discussed. Keeping such a secret from the partner is another betrayal of her.

Most therapy is scheduled at least twice monthly but ideally more often. Not only is it easier to remember the details of the patient's life when meetings are frequent, but the subtle resistances to improvement can be perceived, labeled, and understood more efficiently. To the extent that effective treatment can be short-term, the therapy must carefully maintain its focus on performance anxiety, the triggers for the impotence, and its developmental meanings.

At the end of the evaluation, men need to hear that the therapist feels that there is hope for symptom resolution. When treatment is proving inefficient and ineffective, the patient or couple need the therapist's sustaining optimism even more. This time, however, it must be tempered with the understanding of the nature of the specific psychological obstacles. It is one matter to grasp the nature of a man's intrapsychic problem; it is entirely another matter to work it through. Working through takes time.

Therapists often lose hope faster than patients when they fail to appreciate the time required to work through psychological conflicts. Discouraged patients often respond with hope when the therapist summarizes the forces that have converged to produce the problem.

Sensate Focus Exercises

Sensate focus is a powerful tool for the elimination of performance anxiety. Its essence is the prohibition of intercourse. If the man is willing to follow the therapist's instructions, he will finally be able to relax and concentrate on sensation for the first time since the symptom began. These instructions can be simply given as a suggestion to make love for several weeks without intercourse,[9] or can be elaborately given as described by Masters and Johnson. They reported taking the couple through stages of physical intimacy that always included body touching: first without access to breasts and genitals; then with breast stimulation; then with genital stimulation; then with quiet containment of the penis in the vagina; then with intercourse.

There are three recurring problems with sensate focus exercises. Inexperienced therapists tend to think that these exercises are the treatment. Sensate focus exercises are the tool that the therapist uses to both allay performance anxiety and to determine whose conflicts are standing in the way of lovemaking. Experienced therapists sometimes forget that their dutiful patients are still following the set of instructions given weeks ago. In the rush to understand the resistances, therapists must be careful not to lose track of where the couple is with their assignments. People can be demoralized if they fail to get consistent erections during their "homework." It is best to prescribe sensate focus when the therapist has reason to think that it will restore erections during noncoital lovemaking.

Useful Ideas

Therapy occurs between the therapist and the patient, as well as within the mind of the patient. What the therapist says, how it is said, what it means to the patient, and how it impacts upon his psychic life are all related but distinct phenomena. The mechanisms of therapeutic success are never quite understood; the therapist is never certain what is heard and when, if ever, it will have an impact upon the patient.

There are a few succinctly stated ideas that seem to be helpful for men with potency problems. Each of these has the capacity to jar and educate because these ideas challenge their beliefs about the sexual universe.

"The penis is attached to the heart." Many men believe that their sexual organ is not related to their emotional state. They think of it as an autonomous machine.

"Trying to be a rooster in a hen house, eh!" Many impotent men have trouble with their sexual polygamy even though they have longed for the opportunity.

"I think your penis knows something that you don't." This alerts the patient to the wisdom and self-protecting aspects of his symptom. Another way of saying this is, "This limp penis of yours is your friend. Let's try to figure out how it is trying to help you."

"The penis is the organ of attachment." To the extent that men think of their penises as recreational organs they underestimate the power of intercourse to create an internal emotional connection to the partner in both the man and the woman.

"You, like almost everyone else making love for the first time with a partner, are engaged in a two-horse race: Fear is running against Excitement." This counters the notion that the patient is the only man who has anxiety about intercourse.

"I think you will eventually be fine!" When therapists can honestly say this, they should, because it sustains the man's hope.

BIOLOGICAL THERAPIES

There are four modern physical interventions available for men with impotence: penile prostheses, intracorporal injections of vasodilating substances, vacuum pumps, and medications. The first three are primarily used for organic and mixed impotence. Recently, experience has been accumulating about the use of biological therapies for psychogenic impotence. Medications are used for mixed and psychogenic impotence.

Penile Prostheses

It is well within the technical competence of most urologists to implant a manufactured device within the corpora cavernosa that will restore the mechanical capacity to conduct intercourse. The technology of penile prostheses has been evolving since the early 1950s, but achieved widespread usage beginning in the 1970s. Prostheses fall into two major categories: the types that have a flaccid and erect state and those that maintain a state of semirigidity. Many organically impaired men reject this treatment because it involves hospitalization and surgery and carries a moderate risk of mechanical failure that necessitates reoperation—perhaps one in four patients during the first 5 postoperative years.

Intracorporal Injections

Since the middle 1980s, experience has been accumulating with home injection programs. Men are instructed in how to use a small syringe and needle to inject vasodilating substances directly in a corpus cavernosum. These substances—papaverine, phentolamine, and prostaglandin E^1— produce an erection within 30 minutes which is more than adequate for intercourse. By adjusting the dose, duration can be changed. Injections are effective in cases of mild and moderate arterial insufficiency, sinusoidal dysfunction, neurogenic, and psychogenic impotence. They are ineffective in severe arterial insufficiency and venous leakage. Men with neurogenic impotence are particularly susceptible to priapism with these substances due to end-organ hypersensitivity. Physicians need to provide lower doses to the neurally impaired. The problems with the injections are: about half of impotent men reject the idea of self-injection even though it is not particularly painful; prolonged use can result in nodule formation, which carries the risk of penile curvatures; people with tremors or poor visual acuity are not able to inject themselves and require continued medical supervision.

Vacuum Pumps

In the last several years, many men have been electing to use an external hand-held vacuum device to elicit erections. This plastic system consists of a cylinder into which the flaccid penis is placed, and on which is rolled a rubber band. A short plastic tube connects the cylinder to a light-weight vacuum pump. A sealant is applied to the opening of the cylinder so that a good airtight seal is achieved between the cylinder and the abdominal wall. The man squeezes the handle of the pump which causes the air pressure around the penis to lower. This forces blood into the penis. The pumping continues for several minutes until a long and circumferentially enlarged erection is formed. The rubber band is rolled onto the base of the penis in order to restrict venous return. The erection, not usually as rigid as with the prostheses or injections, persists for about half an hour. The rubber band is removed at the end of intercourse and the penis returns to a flaccid state.

A number of companies make a vacuum pump. Patients' acceptance is much higher than with the prostheses or injections. A one-time investment to purchase the system, the lack of need for medical follow-up, and the absence of significant complications are contributing to the popularity of these devices. The pump seems to work well regardless of organic etiology, although there are some men who for unclear reasons cannot obtain an adequate erection with this approach. Since the studies of patients who have used one of these three approaches (and occasionally their wives) have shown about similar effectiveness rates—between 80% and 90%— physicians and therapists may simply provide the options and a clear view of the complications and advantages of each method and allow the man and his partner to decide.

Medications

A careful medical evaluation of men with impotence is necessary in order to diagnose underlying illnesses and to ensure that those illnesses previously known are adequately treated. For many decades, testosterone, by mouth or by injection, has been prescribed for psychogenic impotence. This practice is slowing down because testosterone is no better than placebo, may accelerate the growth of occult prostatic cancer, and often increase sex drive without enhancing potency. It has been replaced by yohimbine, a drug which may have slight positive impact on erection but which is usually used as a placebo for men who need to take something to quell their performance anxiety by feeling the drug is helping.

Experimental Surgery

Reports repeatedly appear about two new surgical approaches to organic impotence: revascularization of the penis by bringing other arteries into the penis in various locations; and venous ligation for venous leakage. The reasons that these procedures are labeled "experimental" are that they have not yet been convincingly demonstrated to work well, the initial good responses do not last, and other surgeons cannot replicate the good clinical findings.

TED—A CASE HISTORY

Ted became impotent at 50 when he became a cuckold. It was shocking to hear the story of this well-educated upper-class man who had been a star at everything he had tried. He was robust, successful, handsome, athletic, kind, intelligent, generous, and devoutly Christian. He and his wife were building their dream home. During his preoccupation with a year-long business crisis and the back-to-back deaths of his father and uncle, he had not noticed that his wife and the architect were spending inordinate amounts of time together. When he discovered it, he asked her to go to marital therapy, hoping that she would come to her senses. During therapy, she made it clear that she was unwilling to give up the relationship. Within several months, his willingness to stay married was lost. He continued with the marital therapist to process his devastation and soon to deal with his children's reactions to the loss of their parents' marriage. Therapy was helpful; eventually he became engaged and discovered that in the 3 years since his last intercourse, he had become impotent. He could not work out the problem with his own psychotherapist or in brief conjoint therapy with another one during the first 2 years of marriage. Now that he was 53, his only erections were transient, less than rigid, and occurred in the morning once every several months. A physician suggested that he have a prosthesis implanted since he seemed to have a form of organic impotence, PBI=0.7. He said he did not feel ready for it.

At our 2-hour psychiatric evaluation, I told him that it seemed that he, an angerless man, worshipped at the altar of reason, and that his penis knew something about his feelings that he did not. After three emotionally powerful psychotherapy sessions, during which he elaborated upon his struggle to be fair with the settlement so as not to further limit his children's opportunities, his father's infidelity when Ted was 12, the extreme goodness of fit with his new wife, and his extended family's dependence upon him, he reported the presence of good, though transient, erections with his wife. I encouraged him to compose a "letter" to his ex-wife to express what he thought about her behavior, and to do it in a style that reflected his earthy humanity rather than his cultured, analytic rationality. One paragraph from his eight pages of compelling prose follows:

> I despise you for desecrating me as a person and everything I worked for and stood for all of my life. In the vernacular, you are a BITCH, a JERK, and ASSHOLE. My vocabulary of profane and vulgar descriptors is somewhat limited, so let's just leave it that you are a TURKEY TURD! But don't be so naive as to believe that my anger goes only as deep as a few expletives. No, my rage goes to the depths of my intellect and to the heights of my emotion. You are too shallow to comprehend the full extent of the fury your cruelty has ignited, but some day you will come to understand your own petty insignificance when you see yourself as a grovelling turkey turd looking up at soaring eagles gliding in noble and loving skies of peace and joy.

After several weeks of better intercourse and occasional failures, Ted's erectile capacity disappeared. I suggested that his anger at his first wife continued to be a part of the problem. "I understand, but I don't feel it!" Months later, while snow-plowing, his plow landed in a ditch and he responded with uncharacteristic rage. "Where did it come from?" he wondered. Later in the session, he spoke of his frustration about his new wife's refusal to stick to the budget they had agreed upon. He was devoted to building up his estate for her, while she preferred to live to the hilt now. This focus did not help his erections, which were occasionally present. Secure potency followed 3 months later when we discussed his morality, his father's ladies' man behavior, and his adolescent determination to disgrace his father by being the finest human being possible.

Although Ted's performance anxiety was strong, his gender identity was relatively intact because the rest of his life was so successful. The precipitant, his first wife's infidelity, not only created an array of feelings that he suppressed, but it also stirred up his feelings about his inept, morally reprehensible father. Ted's ability to think his way through life contributed to the mystery of his impotence. The ability of the therapist to have him feel the impact of his being a cuckold, a divorced father, an irritated new husband, and an enraged morally superior son enabled his potency to return.

This formulation, based on 15 hours of therapy, sometimes spaced 3 weeks apart, is not necessarily complete or correct. I expect that other therapists would phrase Ted's psychodynamics differently. It is possible that the key elements that maintained the problem were never identified.

The problem with psychological pathogenesis is that one is never certain one has the full story.

SUMMARY

Erectile dysfunction arises from diverse causes and increases in prevalence by each decade, especially after age 50. A man complaining of erectile dysfunction can be diagnostically assigned to one of four categories—psychogenic, organic, mixed, and idiopathic—by using clinical methods that begin with history taking from the man and his partner. If still necessary, a physical examination, laboratory studies, and more specialized tests can then be carried out. Diagnosis is reached by integrating information about the pattern of erections, the social circumstances preceding the problem, and findings from the medical workup. A specific etiology is ascertained, if possible, before a treatment recommended is made.

Mental health professionals are expected have realistic, sophisticated views of the processes that produce lifelong and recent-onset psychogenic impotence. Therapists are also assumed to be able to help men to appreciate and work through the emotional dilemmas that prevent reliable sexual functioning. These stem from childhood developmental problems in lifelong impotence and more recent psychological processes in recent-onset impotence. Help for recent-onset impotence may be facilitated by sensate focus exercises, but individual or couples psychotherapy is more commonly necessary to accomplish this goal.

The modern therapeutic armamentarium for erectile problems includes various psychotherapies, placebolike medication, and mechanical erection assistance through the use of vacuum devices, intracorporal injections, or a prosthesis. Although most men who use mechanical assistance have varieties of organic or mixed impotence, these technologies can occasionally be helpful in psychogenic problems that have proven refractory to psychotherapy.

REFERENCES

1. Krane RJ, Goldstein I, De Tejada IS: Impotence. *New England Journal of Medicine*, 1989; 321(24):1648–1659.
2. Thase ME, Reynolds CF, Glanz LM, *et al*: Nocturnal penile tumescence in depressed men. *American Journal of Psychiatry*, 1987; 144:89–92.
3. Schiavi RC: Nocturnal penile tumescence in the evaluation of erectile disorders: A critical review. *Journal of Sex and Marital Therapy*, 1988; 14(2):83–97.
4. Bradley WE, Timm GW, Gallagher JM, Hohnson BK: New method for continuous measurement of nocturnal penile tumescence and rigidity. *Urology*, 1985; 26:4–9.

5. Anders EK, Bradley WE, Krane RJ: Nocturnal penile rigidity measured by the snap-gauge band. *Journal of Urology,* 1983; 129:964–966.
6. Goldstein I: Vasculogenic impotence: Its diagnosis and treatment. In: deVere, White, eds. *Problems in Urology: Sexual Dysfunction.* Philadelphia, JB Lippincott, 1987, pp 547–563.
7. Schiavi R, Schreiner-Engel P, Mandeli J, *et al*: Healthy aging and male sexual function. *American Journal of Psychiatry,* 1990; 147(6):766–771.
8. Levine SB, Risen CB, Althof SE: An essay on the diagnosis and nature of paraphilia. *Journal of Sex and Marital Therapy.* 16(2):89–102, 1990.
9. Hunter, J: *Treatise on Venereal Disease.* London, Mr. G. Nicole and Mr. J. Johnson, 1788, pp. 203–204.

CHAPTER 11

Paraphilia, Dissociation, and Sexual Abuse

We are only now discovering the extent of sexual abuse of children. We are only now beginning to sense the adult sexual and emotional consequences of not protecting the young from overwhelming physical intimacies.

Society in the United States has discovered sexual abuse during the last decade. Research and the media have broadly addressed the large extent of abuse of girls and women. It has been realized that boys, too, are frequently victimized. Initially, this information provoked shock among disbelieving professionals and laypersons. Privacy used to effectively shroud us from such matters as incest, child molestation, sexual harassment, rape, date rape, and other behaviors that confirm the potential dangerousness of sexuality. The sexual abuse of the young is now considered a public health problem rather than an oddity of human experience.

THE LANGUAGE PROBLEM

Sexual offenders, perpetrators, paraphilics, sexual deviants, sexual addicts, sexual compulsives, incest offenders, and *perverts* are the terms used to refer to those whose sexual interests and behaviors offend socially acceptable norms. Unfortunately, there is little professional consistency in the use of these terms. This, therefore, is how I use them.

Paraphilia is a disorder of the intention component of sexual identity. Currently, it is an official DSM-III-R psychiatric diagnosis for a mental illness that leads to unusual and often socially destructive behaviors, such as sex with children, rape, exhibitionism, voyeurism, sexual touching of strangers, masochism, sadism, obscene phone calling, and the like. Specific criteria have to be met to make this diagnosis. Although paraphilia is occasionally diagnosed in women, the term has a male conceptual bias.

Sexual deviance denotes social disapproval of a person's sexual behavior or interests and connotes that the sexuality in focus is socially abnormal. Most paraphilias can easily be included under the umbrella of sexual deviance, but all deviance is not motivated by one of the paraphilias. The degree of social disapproval varies with the degree of victimization. Sexual deviance is easily incorporated into meaning any sexual behavior of which a particular speaker disapproves. For example, professionals who consider homoeroticism and homosexual behavior to be abnormal refer to these patterns as sexual deviance. The specific behaviors that are viewed as deviant vary from culture to culture and from one era to another within the same culture. For instance, those who enjoyed oral-genital sexual stimulation were considered deviants by the mental health establishment in the early decades of this century.

Sexual addiction refers to compulsive sexual behaviors with partners, prostitutes, or pornography or involving masturbation. This recently coined term derives from self-help movements modeled after Alcoholics Anonymous (AA) treatment formats—Sexaholics Anonymous (SA), Sex and Love Addicts (SLA). People who label themselves as sexual addicts usually describe an internal pressure to behave sexually which is experienced as compulsive, driven, or out of control. *Sexual addiction* is not used in the DSM-III-R. Many of the people who describe themselves as sexual addicts have alcohol, substance abuse, or other forms of addictive behaviors. The concept of sexual addiction is not as male oriented as paraphilia, and women are sometimes present in these self-help groups.

Sexual offender refers to people who commit sexual acts that are specifically prohibited by law. A child molester is a criminal, but a man who negotiates to touch, gaze at, or smell a foot for his arousal is not.

Incest offenders are those people who behave sexually with children in their families or stepfamilies. Incest offenders could easily be called sex offenders, sexual deviants, and occasionally sexual addicts, but they are not paraphilic unless the incest is generated by paraphilic mechanisms. Although most incest offenders are fathers or stepfathers of the victims, some are siblings. Mothers and stepmothers can be incest offenders as well.

Sexual perversion is the oldest term in this group of labels; it has appeared as a psychiatric diagnosis throughout the twentieth century. The term has been widely appropriated in language and carries with it the strong connotations of evil and sin. Among nonprofessionals, it refers to people with unusual sexual behaviors and is used in both a whimsical name-calling informality and a serious problem-denoting manner.

PARAPHILIA

Paraphilia has been recognized by psychiatry since 1905.[1] Accounts of paraphilic behaviors have been in various literatures for centuries, however. Freud thought of the paraphilias as deviations in the aim of the sexual instinct. He considered the normal adult aim was to want to unite the penis and the vagina in intercourse. He chose the term *paraphilia* from the Greek words for along the side (*para*) and love (*philia*) for the preferences for sexual behaviors that led to other forms of orgasmic attainment.

The psychoanalytic concept of paraphilia is broad. Paraphilia is discussed in three contexts: the occasional role that unusual sexual behaviors play in many nonparaphilic people's erotic and sexual lives; the sublimation of paraphilic interests into artistic creativity and vocational activities; and the disorders called paraphilias. Today, there is more interest, even among psychoanalysts, in the narrower concept of the disorder.

The paraphilias, the striking variations in what individuals want to do with a sexual partner and what they want the partner to do with them during sexual behavior, occur among heterosexuals, homosexuals, and bisexuals and among those with conventional and unconventional gender identities. A homosexual exhibitionist is paraphilic on the basis of his genital exposures and not on the basis of his erotic responses to males. A transsexual who desires to be beaten during arousal is paraphilic on the basis of masochism and not on the basis of his wish to live as a woman.

The Characteristics of Paraphilia

When a patient is diagnosed as a paraphilic, three attributes are usually present:

1. A longstanding unusual erotic preoccupation that is highly arousing
2. A pressure to act upon the erotic fantasy
3. A sexual dysfunction involving desire, arousal, or orgasm with the partner during conventional sexual behavior

Paraphilia is invariably characterized by the first of these attributes, is typically characterized by the second, and is often characterized by the third.

First Criterion

Erotic intentions are labeled *disordered* when their themes are unusual in content, longstanding in duration, and powerful in arousal. When erotic intentions demonstrate less than these three characteristics, they may be problematic in some way, but they are *not* clearly paraphilic. The *sine qua non* of the diagnosis of paraphilia is unusual, often hostile, dehumanized eroticism which has occupied the patient for most of his adolescent and adult life. This fantasy is often associated with preoccupying arousal when it occurs in daydreams, masturbation fantasies, or is encountered in explicit films or magazines.

From person to person, paraphilic imagery is variable in content, but both the imagined behavior and its implied relationship to the partner are unusual. Paraphilic fantasies are usually preoccupied with aggression. Images of rape, obscene phone calling, exhibitionism, and the touching of strangers, for example, are rehearsals of victimization. In masochistic images, the aggression is directed at the self—autoerotic strangulation, slavery, torture, and spanking. In others, the aggression is well disguised as love of children or teenagers. Aggression is so apparent in most paraphilic content, however, that when none seems to exist, the clinician needs to wonder whether it is absent or hidden. Sadistic, masochistic, exhibitionistic, fetishistic, voyeuristic, or pedophilic fantasies often rely heavily upon the image of a partner who does not possess personhood. Some imagery, in fact, has no pretense of a human partner at all; with clothing, animals, or excretory products being the focus. Other themes, such as the preoccupation with feet or hair, combine both human and inanimate interests.

A person's paraphilic themes may change from time to time. Whether this is actually a shift to a different paraphilia or an elaboration of an existing one is often difficult to ascertain. The shift from imagining talking "dirty" on the phone in order to scare a woman to imagining raping a woman can be considered a new paraphilia or an intensification of sadism. Switches between sadism and masochism and voyeurism and exhibitionism have long been recognized, but changes from voyeurism to pedophilia and from pedophilia to rape have only been recently recognized. For some paraphilics the most significant shifts are from erotic imagery to sexual behavior. Since the triggers for shifts are often inapparent, it is important to keep open the possibility that paraphilia may be a basic disorder with numerous erotic and sexual manifestations.

The use of the adjective "unusual" for paraphilic eroticism creates a slight dilemma. Not only is what is unusual for one clinician not for another, but such paraphilic imagery is by no means rare. Alternative words, such as strange, bizarre, inhuman, and dehumanizing, are not clear improvements. Paraphilic images often involve arousal without the pretense of caring or human attachment. They are images of hatred, anger, fear, vengeance, or worthlessness which often require no familiarity with the partner—they are lustful aggressive images. Paraphilic images are completely conscious and should not be confused with speculations about the unconscious aggression or sadomasochism that some theoreticians assume are part of all sexual behavior.[2]

Most paraphilic adults, even those in their 60s, can trace their fantasy themes to puberty, and many can remember these images from grade school years. When adolescent rapists or incest offenders are evaluated, they often are able to report prepubertal aggressive erotic preoccupations. Men who report periodic paraphilic imagery interspersed with more usual eroticism have had their paraphilic themes from childhood or early adolescence.

Paraphilic fantasies are the key to the man's lustful arousal. When these images are conjured up, the patient can become immediately and intensely aroused. They preoccupy him and, if desired, can quickly lead to orgasm. Many patients describe their arousal as intrusive—that is, as occurring even when it is unwanted. When the paraphilic's themes are encountered in magazines, videotapes, pictures, or over the phone, arousal quickly occurs.[3]

Second Criterion

> For forty years, Jon has masturbated to images of barely clad women violently wrestling each other. Periodically throughout his marriage, he has tried to involve his wife in wrestling matches with her friends and eventually with their adolescent daughter.

The second criterion for the diagnosis is the man's sense that the erotic imagery exerts a pressure on him to play out the scene he imagines. In its milder forms, the pressure results merely in a preoccupation with a behavior; in its more intense forms, it is described as a drivenness to act out the fantasy in sexual *behavior* by oneself or with a partner.

> On occasion when Jon was drunk, he embarrassed his wife by trying to pick fights between her and other women. Socially, he occasionally jokingly suggested that the women wrestle. During much of his sober life, however, his daydreams of women wrestling were private experiences that only preoccupied him. He amassed a collection of magazines and videotapes depicting women wrestling to which he felt driven by the need for excitement.

The usual avenue for discharge of this pressure is masturbation. Frequent masturbation, often more than daily, continues long after adolescence. In the most severe situations, the need to attend to the fantasy and masturbate is so overpowering that life's ordinary activities cannot efficiently occur. Masturbation and sometimes partner-seeking behavior—such as finding a woman to shock through exhibiting an erection—is experienced as driven. The patient reports either that he cannot control his behavior or that he controls it with such great effort that his work, study, parenting, and relationships are disrupted.

This pressure to behave sexually often leads the man to believe he has a high sex drive. So many paraphilics have described their masturbation-to-orgasm frequencies as 10 to 15/day that this may be the upper limit of male sexual capacity. Even when these patients' estimate of their frequency of orgasm strains credulity less, however, the return of sexual drive manifestations soon after orgasm suggests that something is wrong either with these patients' sexual drives or their satiety mechanisms.

A minority of men with paraphilic imagery manage to contain the impulse to attain orgasm for long periods of time. The pressure to masturbate using the imagery only arises when they are not otherwise preoccupied. These patients tend to be perceived as having high ego strength. The DSM-III-R distinguishes mild, moderate, and severe paraphilia on the basis of the ability to contain the sexual urge: those with the mild form never act out the urge; those with the moderate form occasionally have acted out; and those with severe paraphilia repeatedly act out the urge. But the DSM-III-R is assuming that acting out means with a partner. The lives of many "mild" cases are profoundly disrupted by their need to masturbate a dozen times a day without involving a partner.

Masturbation is often not the sole expression of nonvictimizing sexual acting out, of course. Paraphilic men often report collections of pornography that aid their masturbation, frequent visits to sexual book stores to see movies or peep shows, continual use of prostitutes for their special sexual behaviors, or the extensive use of telephone sex.

Victimization of others, the public health problem, is the least common form of sexual acting out but it is by no means rare, as police departments and research studies testify.[4] Exhibitionism, pedophilia, and sadism lead to frequent victimization of strangers.

Third Criterion

A severe sexual dysfunction involving desire, arousal, or orgasm with a partner when the paraphilia conditions are not met can be as striking as the first two criteria. The wives of paraphilics tell stories with these themes: "He is not interested in sex with me." "He never initiates." "He doesn't seem to enjoy our sexual life together except when. . . . " "He is usually not potent." "Even when we do make love, he rarely ejaculates." Research has also documented that the sexual functioning of paraphilic men is significantly poorer than the general population.[5]

> Jon presented for help with his inability to maintain his erection with his wife for intercourse. With the exception of procreational sex, he was not able

to consummate his long marriage. He was able to erect if his wife described that she was wrestling other women while he stimulated his penis in front of her, but he always lost his erection when intercourse was attempted.

This criterion cannot be used as a criterion for diagnosis because many patients do not currently have a sexual partner, some men never have been able to form a relationship with a consenting partner, or only have had the most fleeting sexual behavior with a partner. And there are some paraphilic men who do not have any sexual dysfunction with their partner*. Abel has written that most paraphilics can engage in ordinary sexual behavior without paraphilic imagery,[6] reminding clinicians that sample selection factors inapparently shape the descriptions of psychiatric disorders.

Sexual dysfunction may occur because some paraphilic men have no erotic script for ordinary sexual life. They need their paraphilic fantasy during lovemaking to feel aroused. This preoccupation with something other than what is occurring between the partners precludes a strong sense of emotional connection, which may soon be felt by the partner. These men fear psychological intimacy because it makes them feel the anxiety or dread of being vulnerable to another human being. The paraphilic fantasy is used as an anxiety-reducing technique.

What Is the Nature of the Problem with Paraphilia?

Abel recognized paraphilia as an impairment in the bonding function of sexuality. Freund and Blanchard[7] classified it as a courtship disorder. Stoller[3] thought paraphilia represented the erotic form of hatred—a hatred motivated by the need for revenge for childhood trauma. Fenichel and Freud thought that this disorder represented the fixations to their childhood thoughts that women had penises (phallic women) and that they were in danger of losing theirs (castration anxiety). Cooper posited that paraphilics share a core set of dynamics involving the unsuccessful repair of early life experiences with a terrifying, malignant, malicious mother—their problem is that they have not been able to survive their passive, helpless experiences with their preoedipal mothers.[8] Paraphilics tend to equate women with their internal image of their frightening mothers. Kaplan recently emphasized the view that paraphilia is a strategy to stabilize masculine or feminine gender identity. Paraphilic strategies attempt to deny the differences between the sexes and the generations of child and parents.[9]

---

*Many potent men think of themselves as normal because their penises erect and ejaculate. They do not consider their lack of satiety, evidenced by a reactivation of the need for sexual behavior soon after orgasm with a partner, to be a sign of dysfunction. As this is a matter of interpretation by the therapist as well, the point is debatable.

Every idea in the previous paragraph is probably partially correct. Paraphilics have a significant multidimensional problem. They have a sexual identity disorder that makes erotic normality impossible to attain. Culture asks us to have some image of attachment, some ability to neutralize anger toward others, to contain the anxiety over closeness, and to emotionally want to simultaneously enhance the self and the partner through sexual contact. Ordinary intentions aim for peaceable mutuality between real people, paraphilic ones aim at aggressive one-sidedness. This sexual identity disorder could be referred to as a masculinity disorder except that it occasionally occurs in women.

Paraphilia is also a disorder of self-regulation in which there is an enigmatic paradox between what one wants to be and what one is. Paraphilia leaves the person with a hunger for a behavior which often feels uncontrollable or sick. This hunger paradox usually has profound effects on the person's internal experience because these problems rob the person of autonomy. This is why it is often thought of as an addiction.

> A 33-year-old, religious, married mother of two sought help for depression with chronic suicidal ideation, tranquilizer abuse, and aversion to sexual behavior with her loved husband. She had been masturbating to masochistic imagery almost every day of her life since age four. She easily attained orgasm through images of being pierced, penetrated, burned, medically instrumented, or otherwise tortured, but became physically ill when her husband touched her. As she was promoted within a religious institution to positions of higher visibility and great responsibility, her desperation about her inability to live the life she wanted became less tolerable to her and her drug abuse increased.

Paraphilia is also a disorder of the capacity to love. It permanently delays the evolution from adolescent lustful, impersonal erotic images to adult person-to-person imagery. The paraphilic person cannot allow the partner to be both a source of affectionate connection and physical pleasure.

The Scientific Measurement Process

The previous descriptions of paraphilia derive from clinical evaluations and psychotherapies. There is another emerging line of description about male sex offenders that adds to the understanding of paraphilia. Erectile responses to visual stimulation in the laboratory began to be studied in the early 1960s.[10] During the next two decades, scientific work was done exploring the validity of reliability of penile responses to fantasies, slides, audiotapes, and videotapes as a means of evaluating child molesters and rapists. This work aimed to devise a standardized assessment protocol so that clinical evaluation could move beyond self-report data to make clinical judgments about potentially dangerous men.

Early studies were able to distinguish pedophilic from nonpedophilic responses to still pictures of children, adolescents, and adults. They demonstrated that, as a group, nonfamilial child molesters (pedophiles) experience greater arousal to children than nonoffenders and also show substantial arousal to adults. Although incestuous men, as a group, do not show pedophilic responses, their responses to adults are midway between the pedophiles and the normals.[11] When audiotapes that varied the aggression content were used, some of the distinctions between incestuous and nonfamilial offenders became less clear. The laboratory can also distinguish homosexual from heterosexual pedophiles.

Later, more methodologically sophisticated work identified five profiles from the phallometric responses to visual and auditory stimulation:

1. "Adult"—strong responses to females who are 20 years old+; moderate responses to 16–18-year-olds; minimal responses to females less than 15 years old.
2. "Teen–adult"—strong responses to females who are 13 years old+; decreasing responses to younger people.
3. "Nondiscriminating"—moderate responses to all ages.
4. "Child–adult"—strong responses to both females 18 years+ and to those 11 years and younger with weak responses to 12–14-year-olds.
5. "Child"—strong responses to those 11 years and younger with weak responses to those 13 years and older.

Seventy percent of nonoffenders had an "adult" profile, while the remainder had either a "teen–adult" or "nondiscriminating" pattern. Forty percent of incest offenders had an "adult" profile, 40% had a "nondiscriminating" profile, and almost 20% had a "teen–adult" profile. None had a "child" profile. Nonfamilial child molesters, whether they targeted male or female children, were heterogeneous in their patterns: 35% had a "child" profile; the rest were equally distributed among the four other profiles.[12] Pedophiles, therefore, should not be thought of as necessarily having exclusive responses to children.

A number of studies have shown that rapists respond both to adult visual cues and violent nonconsenting audio cues, whereas normals respond to adult cues and only minimally to nonconsenting ones. The ability to make these distinctions increases markedly when the assessment is done a second time.[13] Phallometric studies have suggested that rapists and child molesters who have been more violent with their victims respond more to violent stimuli in the laboratory.

Phallometric studies of adolescent sex offenders have shown that those who were sexually abused demonstrate more sexual arousal to visual stimuli than offenders who were not.[14]

Science is likely to continue to make contributions both to the clinical assessment of paraphilics and offenders and to the emergence of a theory about the pathogenesis of unusual eroticism and sexuality. This line of work constantly reminds dynamically oriented clinicians that it is not entirely safe to make generalizations about all paraphilics. Sex-offending paraphilics are a heterogeneous group.[15] The work also never allows scientists to forget how difficult it is to establish a finding as a fact.[16]

DISSOCIATION

In ordinary states of consciousness, the brain integrates our experiences and produces a continuity of identity, memory, and time. The discontinuities of these dimensions of experience, when they are not produced by other major psychopathologies, are referred to as *dissociation*. Dissociative phenomena range from the nearly universal, normal, temporary use of defenses when bad news is heard to much less frequent, profound psychopathologies—such as posttraumatic stress disorder, fugue and amnesia states, and multiple personality disorder.

The capacity to dissociate, while everpresent, is maximal during childhood. Children who were exposed to overwhelming physical or emotional trauma, especially sexual abuse, retain the capacity for easy dissociation in response to stress far longer than those who were not traumatized. In childhood, situations that produce overwhelming pain, fear, or helplessness may be automatically reacted to with dissociative defenses, which create the illusion for the child of controlling the out-of-control situation. The child detaches and has subjective experiences consisting of derealization, depersonalization, perceptions that the beating or sexual stimulation is happening to someone else, a numbing of all sensation, or a dazed state of shock. Similar reactions have been repeatedly seen among adults whose lives have been in sudden danger—such as in a natural disaster, rape, a collapse of a building, or combat. Symptoms that follow such trauma do not quickly disappear once the danger has passed. Memory, perception, time sense, concentration, flashbacks, and other discontinuities of ordinary consciousness continue.

Dissociation is a helpful concept in understanding the consequences of sexual abuse, the subjective experiences of paraphilics, how ordinary arousal differs from paraphilic arousal, and what males with paraphilia and females with multiple personality disorder may have in common.

Multiple Personality Disorder and Sexual Abuse

Although sexual abuse is not the only overwhelming trauma to facilitate the development of this dramatic, no longer rare disorder, almost all patients with multiple personality disorder (MPD) allege incestuous sexual abuse during their childhoods.[17,18] Although the abuse histories are often severe, bizarre, and subject to the distortions of remote memory, efforts to independently corroborate these histories have been successful.[19] Given estimates of sexual abuse of females that range up to 62%, it is likely that MPD either is an unusual outcome of sexual abuse or that it is an outcome when the abuse is particularly brutal, longlasting, and associated with other continuing inadequacies of nurturance and protection.

Patients with MPD carry many other diagnoses, have numerous symptoms, and usually do not improve unless the nature of the problem is accurately perceived. They are notoriously difficult to diagnose—the average patient is misdiagnosed for approximately 6 years. I consider MPD to be a model for the worst case outcome of childhood sexual abuse. Lesser degrees of dissociative symptomatology with various disorders of anxiety, depression, sexual function, and substance abuse are probably far more frequent.

Provera, Paraphilia, and Dissociation

In the early 1980s, depo-Provera began to be used to treat paraphilics who were either constantly masturbating, seeking out personally dangerous sexual outlets, or committing sex crimes. The weekly injections (400 to 600 mg) were often dramatically successful: the men reported being able to work, study, or participate in activities that previously were beyond them because of concentration or attention difficulties.[20] In the late 1980s, the oral form of Provera (medroxy-progesterone) began to be administered in doses ranging from 30 mg to 80 mg/day with similar results: men reported a better sense of integration. They could attend to their real problems and no longer felt they were living in a time warp in which their sexual needs took priority over other life demands—and they did not have the weight gain, hypertension, muscle cramps, and gynecomastia that those on injections experienced. Even though paraphilic patients frequently spoke of trancelike erotic preoccupations, loss of time, and fuzzy memory for what they had done, clinicians generally have not perceived their symptoms as dissociative phenomena.

> Thirty-three-year-old Ben sought help after a man he picked up in the park forced him to wear a belt tightly around his neck while the patient was anally raped. This near-asphyxia experience terrified him. Now a clerk, he could not finish college because his masochistic fantasies and relentless arousal kept him from concentrating. His frequent sexual partners had always been strangers. Danger had excited him in his fantasies as long as he could remember and in recent years he was seeking out danger in his sexual behaviors.
>
> When asked about his orientation, he was unsure even though all of his eroticism was directed at men. He complained of the loss of time during his

cruising for partners and living in a haze most of the time. He was not a drug user. He consistently represented his sexual encounters as ego-dystonic. During a year's treatment with depo-Provera, his masturbation decreased from 4–6 times/day to a few times per week. He returned to college, did well in his studies, and emphasized that he now felt gay because "I can choose to be with a man. Before, I wasn't sure what I was!" His masochistic imagery faded considerably.

There is a growing body of clinical experience with paraphilic men that suggests that they have a high incidence of sexual abuse histories, often intrafamilial in nature. Some clinicians quote as high as 85%. However, men find it difficult to admit to sexual abuse, especially by another male, because they often worry that they were chosen because the abuser perceived something unmasculine or "gay" about them. Freund *et al.*, distrusting self-report data of men with criminal histories, conducted a phallometric study that demonstrated at least twice the incidence of sexual abuse among pedophiles than among homosexuals and heterosexuals, but raised doubts as to the trustworthiness of these memories.[21] Even in the face of doubts about the errors in underreporting and the motives for overreporting, it is reasonable to consider that sexual abuse in childhood is one factor that may play an important role in the evolution of paraphilic eroticism. Few psychiatric diagnoses are explained by a single factor.

Alterations of Consciousness during Ordinary Lovemaking

Highly pleasing, nonparaphilic sex between consenting partners results in progressively focused attention on sensation. The partners free their minds from worldly concerns and become one with their skin sensations. Fantasy may appear during the caressing for some, presumably to add to the arousal. Regardless, lovemaking obliterates the sense of time and often creates a sense of drifting off to somewhere else. In some particularly intense loving interactions, men and women also report a loss of ego boundaries in which the partners seem to be one for a few seconds, often as orgasm approaches. These discontinuities of identity and time, which sometimes trigger fantasies or memories of other exciting sexual experiences, are normal. Psychoanalysts sometimes refer to lovemaking as regression in the service of the ego—that is, sometimes giving up the usual state of consciousness produces a highpoint of pleasure.

The appreciation of the normal dissociative aspects of lovemaking helps us to consider two important clinical hypotheses: paraphilic arousal is often a pathological exaggeration of ordinary dissociation; adults who were sexually abused as children may have desire problems because as they dissociate during normal arousal, memories of their abuse threaten to come to consciousness.

The first hypothesis has been emphasized by Stoller[3] who perceives from listening to others talk about their subjective experiences of arousal, that paraphilic arousal is more intense, preoccupying, and pleasurable than arousal described by people without paraphilia. The second hypothesis provides a reasonable motive for withdrawing from the sexual arena for a lifetime and provides an explanation for being comfortable as an asexual person.

SEXUAL ABUSE

What Constitutes Sexual Abuse of Children?

Sexual abuse of children is based on the idea that children cannot legally consent to participate in sexual behavior with an adult, even when they cooperate with the behavior. This is because of the power differential between child and older person and the child's inability to understand the impact of sexual behavior. Society now expects its citizens to protect its children. These legal and social values are no longer controversial.

Scientific studies, which frequently are controversial, rest upon arbitrary definitions. Sexual abuse is typically defined as requiring a 5-year age difference between the child less than age 13 and the sexual partner. Some workers require a 10-year difference between an adolescent and the partner, while others define abuse by nonconsent and coercion regardless of the age of the perpetrator.[22] The behaviors that are considered abusive: kissing, oral-genital stimulation, vaginal, anal, or oral stimulation with a body part or an inanimate object, exhibition of nudity, looking at the child's nude body, taking pictures of the child's naked body, and showing sexually explicit materials to children. These behaviors typically occur in the context of the sexual gratification of the adult. No definition, however, can be expected to capture all sexually abusive situations. The lines between abusive, inappropriate, and acceptable within a particular family cannot always be easily drawn.

How Common Is Sexual Abuse of Children?

Peters *et al.* summarized the range of estimated prevalence of sexual abuse for females as from 6% to 62%; for males the range was exactly half.[23] The studies used different populations and different methods, of course. The figures that are usually quoted are that from 20% to 30% of adult American women have a history of sexual contact between the ages of 5 and 9 years with a person at least 5 years older; once again, men's histories indicate about one-half the prevalence. Among psychiatric inpatients, the prevalence is approximately 50%. In the psychiatric emergency room, the prevalence rises to approximately 70% when patients are carefully asked.[24] The abuse that the women seeking emergency services reported began, on average, at age 8, lasted over 4 years, and involved more than one perpetrator. Intercourse occurred in 74%. Incest occurred in 74%.

The pattern of abuse varies according to sex. Boys tend to be less than 12 when initially abused and are more likely to be abused by another boy outside the family and to be threatened physically.

Effects of Sexual Abuse on Children and Adolescents

The answers to questions about short- and long-term effects of sexual abuse draw dramatic distinctions between clinical impressions and scientific studies. Clinicians, who see sexually abused children or adults tend to assume that although the effects may be varied, they are profound and lasting, not only on adult sexual capacity but on general personality functioning. Scientists point up the methodologic limitations involved in making such conclusions. It is not that those who study this question scientifically strongly disagree with clinicians' opinions. The opposite is probably true; it is just that scientists are being true to their discipline—facts require systematized evaluations of patients and controls and follow-up.

Conte[25] has recently reviewed this topic and has concluded that

> it is clear that sexual abuse is associated with significant mental health problems in childhood and adulthood. Data suggest that not all victims are affected in the same way or to the same extent. For example 21% of the abused children . . . were asymptomatic (p. 294).

One of the consistent findings of sexually abused children is that they are more likely to exhibit sexual behaviors that were generally unseen among normal controls and psychiatric outpatients.[26]

Both clinicians and researchers use the term *sexualized* for the most severely affected children. Depending on their age, sexualized children may masturbate in public, initiate sex with other children, offer themselves sexually to adults, display cross-gender behaviors, or begin to talk incessantly "dirty." These girls and boys are distinctly different from other children. Their behavior, among its other functions, may be motivated by a wish to alert the society to their need for rescue. Nonspecific psychiatric symptoms, such as substance abuse, self-mutilation, eating or sleep disturbances, depression, poor school performance, sociopathy, and somatization, may indirectly signal the presence of sexual abuse. In more recent years, the diagnosis of posttraumatic stress disorder has been thought to encompass the symptomatology following sexual abuse.

Effects of Sexual Abuse on Adults

There are many studies that indicate that there are frequent multidimensional consequences of childhood and adolescent sexual victimization.

Incest survivors, for instance, in a community sample of African- and white American women, have been demonstrated to display patterns of either failure to enjoy sex and subsequent loss of interest in it or a highly active drivenness for sexual experience. Incest survivors are less likely to use birth control, have more unplanned pregnancies and abortions, and remain at risk for sexually transmitted diseases including AIDS; they also have lower self-esteem, poor body images, and have a variety of manifestations of sexual dysfunction.[27,28]

CLINICAL IMPLICATIONS

Hostile Countertransference

Most beginning therapists have strong hostility and disgust reactions to adults who sexually abuse children. These affects usually immediately surface and generally produce a hesitance to be involved clinically. Both sexes are avoidant, but particularly women. Comments such as "Hang him," "Throw the scum in jail," or "Not on your life" are readily elicited when such a case is assigned in general psychiatric settings.

The age-old association between paraphilia (not just sex offenders) and evil is quickly mobilized in the therapist. The therapist who can offer psychiatric evaluation and therapy to paraphilics despite these private reactions may reap these rewards: they can be helpful to many paraphilics and their families; future victimization can be prevented; the therapist has an opportunity to consider the psychology of evil; and the therapist's understanding of erotic and sexual symptom formation may be greatly enhanced. To offer help, however, means that the countertransference must be faced, understood, and respected.

These feelings provide a passionate introduction to the question of whether mental health professionals have any legitimate evaluation and therapeutic role with criminal offenders. Sex offenders are usually dealt with in forensic settings or in specialty clinics that have a workable interacting with lawyers, probation officers, and protective service personnel. Even in these settings, which continue to proliferate because of the recognition of the high prevalence of these problems, there are questions whether the society is better off treating or incarcerating the sex offender. Evidence of the helpfulness of therapeutic intervention for some offenders *per se* is not enough to settle the issue because offenders are continually encountered who are not treatment candidates.

The effects of sexual abuse and paraphilia on character formation has not yet been mentioned. Sometimes, it is apparent that an offender is an obnoxious, dangerous, remorseless man, who denies his culpability even when faced with the evidence of his guilt. Sometimes, a substance-abusing woman is seen whose deterioration has eroded whatever maternal nurturance she used to possess. More often, however, the offender is more perplexing because he seems like an otherwise reasonable human being, who is as much a victim as he is a victimizer. The therapist is forced to confront a range of complex moral, social, and psychiatric issues. Some professionals find this area too confusing, whereas others find the paradoxes and contradictions worthy of personal investment.

Therapists have subjective reactions to abused children that also mirror the general population's attitudes. "This could not have occurred! Things like this don't really happen. It must be her imagination." Or, "The child must have done something to provoke it." Or, "What a disgusting family! Both parents must be at fault. Anyway, it is too complicated a situation for me. Let someone else take care of them." It is far easier to overcome these potentially interfering reactions when the focus is on the victimized children than when it is placed on the perpetrator. The typical organization of psychiatric services, in fact, separates services for the victim and the perpetrator.

The Evaluation and Treatment of the Offender

During the evaluation of sex offenders, the patient should be allowed to tell his story, but it should be responded to with a series of questions that explore the developmental sequence of fantasies and behaviors. Sometimes paraphilia may involve only one deviant activity, but usually two or more are currently present and the man has passed through phases during which other paraphilic imagery and behaviors preoccupied him. It is important that more skepticism be applied to those accused of sex offenses than other patients. Experienced therapists have been lied to so many times that they have become tough questioners. They eventually learn that paraphilia is a long-standing disorder with protean manifestations, often associated with substance abuse and other signs of impaired social functioning. They are far less likely to be taken in by initial presentations than they were when they began this work.

> A 36-year-old cardiologist sought help for another outbreak of obscene phone calling after the police traced his third phone call to the same woman. In his midteens and his twenties, he had several undiscovered periods of obscene phone calls accompanied by masturbation. He quickly linked this activity to his adolescent shyness with girls, his feelings that his body shape and his personality were defective ("I was a nerdy, uncoordinated kid!"), and to a painful refusal of a girl to go on a date with him at age 16.
>
> He was puzzled by his lack of motivation to make love to his wife. He complained of depression since he was identified by the police, and anxiety over the implications of his crime on his medical license. He denied other paraphilic interests. He always was concerned during his therapy about the

time it required to be away from his practice. (He drove two hours to his therapy.) His depression dramatically improved without medication or understanding its dynamics. He began to make love to his wife. Just as there seemed to be little reason for further meetings, he was jailed.

After a program on sexual abuse in her high school, his 16-year-old stepdaughter indicated that she had been her father's sexual partner for 4 years.

When psychotherapies are undertaken, alone or along with androgen-depleting medications, antidepressants, or anticompulsion drugs, the therapist may come to recognize that paraphilic symptoms serve useful purposes in the patient's life. They prevent the recall of poor-quality parental relationships and personal, sexual, physical, and emotional victimization. The symptoms stabilize the patient's sexual identity. Many of these men are privately worried about their orientation or gender identity. Paraphilia shores up a faltering sense of masculinity. The cardiologist only had to worry that he was doing something "wrong" by having intercourse with his stepdaughter; he did not have to worry that he was inadequate as a man.

More dramatic, however, is the observation that the symptoms are a defense against dysphoric feelings. Paraphilic eroticism often is used as a retreat from anxiety, sadness, loneliness, guilt, or anger of whatever source. In a more global way, the symptoms are also a defense against adapting to the demands of life. Paraphilia is a dissociative retreat to a private world instead of dealing with life's challenges. Paraphilics with poor adaptive functioning, in general, may seem almost psychotic in their retreat into compulsive sexual behaviors when life requires a great deal from them, whereas better functioning people may meet their demands, yet only feel as though their eroticism has become too important.

SUMMARY

Ordinary erotic and sexual intentions involve peaceable mutuality between real people. This significant developmental accomplishment rests on four internal mental capacities: to be able to have an image of human attachment; to be able to neutralize anger toward others; to be able to tolerate anxiety over closeness; and to want to enhance the self and the partner through sexual contact. Paraphilia is a sexual identity disorder that aims at aggressive one-sidedness in erotic and sexual life. It represents a critical impairment in the capacity to love.

Dissociation is a defensive capacity employed by children and adults to deal with perceived threats to life and physical comfort. The capacity to dissociate provides an important linkage between sexual abuse of children, paraphilia in adolescents and adults, and the dramatic and more subtle dissociative disorders. These problems are probably etiologically related.

Sexual abuse of children is a national problem of epidemic proportions, so prevalent that it probably plays a role in diverse mental health problems. Among the least well-known consequences of sexual abuse is relentless sexual excitement, only briefly satiated by orgasm. Most sexually compulsive men and women are neither quickly recognized as having a paraphilia nor as having been sexually abused as children.

Therapists can be helpful both to the abused and to the sex offender with a variety of clinical approaches, including those that involve psychodynamic considerations of the role the paraphilic behavior plays in the regulation of their affect states. Two preliminary processes are required, however: the hostile countertransference must be understood, respected, and overcome; and the evaluation must be informed by past experience with offenders who either lie or minimize their accounts of the extent of their sexual crimes.

REFERENCES

1. Freud S: Three essays on the theory of sexuality, in Strachy L (ed): *The Standard Edition of the Complete Works of Sigmund Freud*, Vol 7. London, Hogarth Press (1953) 1905, pp 125–243.
2. Kernberg OF: Aggression and love in the relationship of a couple, in Fogel GI, Myers WA, (eds): *Perversions and Near-Perversions in Clinical Practice: New Psychoanalytic Perspectives.* New Haven, Yale University Press, 1991.
3. Stoller R: *Perversion: The Erotic Form of Hatred.* New York, Pantheon, 1975.
4. Abel GG, Becker JV, Mittelman MS, *et al*: Self-reported sex crimes of nonincarcerated parphiliacs. *Journal of Interpersonal Violence*, 1987; 2–3.
5. Pawlak AE, Boulet JR, Bradford JMW: Discriminant analysis of a sexual-function inventory with intrafamilial and extrafamilial child molesters. *Archives of Sexual Behavior*, 1991; 20(1):27–34.
6. Abel GG: Paraphilias, in Kaplan HI and Sadock BJ (eds): *Comprehensive Textbook of Psychiatry V.* Baltimore, Williams & Wilkins, 1989, pp 1069–1085.
7. Freund K, Blanchard R: The concept of a courtship disorder. *Journal of Sex and Marital Therapy*, 1986; 12(2):79–92.
8. Cooper AM: The unconscious core of perversion, in Fogel GI, Myers WA (eds): *Perversions and Near-Perversions in Clinical Practice: New Psychoanalytic Perspectives.* New Haven, Yale University Press, 1991, pp 17–35.
9. Kaplan LJ: *Female Perversions: The Temptation of Emma Bovary.* New York, Doubleday, 1991.
10. Freund K: A laboratory method of diagnosing predominance of homo- and hetero-erotic interest in the male. *Behaviour Research and Therapy*, 1963; 1:85–93.
11. Quinsey VL, Steinman CM, Bergersen SG, Homes TF: Penile circumference, skin conductance, and ranking responses of child molesters and normals to sexual and nonsexual visual stimuli. *Behavior Therapy*, 1975; 6:213–219.
12. Barbaree HE, Marshall WL: Erectile responses amongst heterosexual child molesters, father-daughter incest offenders and matched nonoffenders: Five distinct age preference profiles. *Canadian Journal of Behavioral Science*, 1989; 21:70–82.
13. Yates E, Barbaree HE, Marshall WL: Anger and deviant sexual arousal. *Behavior Therapy*, 1984; 15:287–294.
14. Becker JV, Hunter JA, Stein RM, Kaplan MS: Factors associated with erection in adolescent sex offenders. *Journal of Psychopathology and Behavioral Assessment*, 1989; 11(4):353–362.

15. Becker JV, Kaplan MS, Tenke CE: The influence of abuse history and denial on erectile response profiles of adolescent sexual perpetrators. *Behavior Therapy,* 1992; 23:87-97.
16. Simon WT, Schouten PGW: Plethysmography in the assessment and treatment of sexual deviance: An overview. *Archives of Sexual Behavior,* 1991; 20(1):75–91.
17. Putnam FW, Guroff JJ, Silberman EK, *et al.*: The clinical phenomenology of multiple personality disorder: Review of 100 recent cases. *Journal of Clinical Psychiatry,* 1986; 47:285–293.
18. Schultz R, Braun BG, Kluft RP: Multiple personality disorder; phenomenology of selected variables in comparison to major depression. *Dissociation,* 1989; 2:45–51.
19. Coons PM, Millstein V: Psychosexual disturbances in multiple personality. *Journal of Nervous and Mental Diseases,* 1986; 47:106–110.
20. Berlin F, Meinecke CF: Treatment of sex offenders with antiandrogenic medication: Conceptualization, review of treatment modalities, and preliminary findings. *American Journal of Psychiatry,* 1981; 138:601–607.
21. Freund K, Watson R, Dickey R: Does sexual abuse in childhood cause pedophilia? An exploratory study. *Archives of Sexual Behavior,* 1990; 19(6):557–567.
22. Wyatt GE: Child sexual abuse and its effects on sexual functioning, in Bancroft J, Davis CM, Ruppel HJ (eds): *Annual Review of Sex Research: An Integrative and Interdisciplinary Review Vol II.* Lake Mills, Iowa, Society for the Scientific Study of Sex, 1991, pp 249–266.
23. Peters SD, Wyatt GE, Finkelhor D: Prevalence, in Finkelhor D (ed): *A Sourcebook on Child Sexual Abuse.* Beverly Hills, Sage, 1986, pp 81–87.
24. Briere J, Zaidi LY: Sexual abuse histories and sequelae in female psychiatric emergency room patients. *American Journal of Psychiatry,* 1990; 146(12): 1602–1606.
25. Conte JR: Overview of child sexual abuse, in Tasman A, Goldfinger SM (eds): *Review of Psychiatry Volume 10.* Washington, D.C., American Psychiatric Press, 1991.
26. Friedrich WN: Behavior problems in sexually abused children: An adaptional perspective, in Wyatt G, Powell G (eds): *Lasting Effects of Child Sexual Abuse.* Newbury Park, CA, Sage, 1988.
27. Wyatt GE, Newcomb M, Riederle M, Notgrass C: *The Effects of Child Sexual Abuse on Women's Sexual Functioning and Psychological Functioning.* Newbury Park, CA., Sage, 1992.
28. Gold ER: Long-term effects of sexual victimization in childhood: An attributional approach. *Journal of Consulting and Clinical Psychology,* 1986; 54:471-475.

CHAPTER 12

Homosexualities

Mental health professionals can get beyond culture's profound fear of and antagonism to homosexual persons, but generally not without effort at learning and self-examination. The personal and clinical rewards are considerable.

There probably is no more passionate controversy within the realm of human sexuality than that stimulated by the men and women who are interested in and behave sexually with members of their own sex. Homosexuality creates anxiety, hatred, moral outrage, soul-searching, debate, and discrimination by most ethnic, age, and political groups. Homosexual imagery, behaviors, and life-styles are deeply upsetting to many individuals and the institutions that they form. Historically, homosexual persons have been frequently designated as the enemy, and occasionally in history the enemy's crime has been considered so treasonous as to be punished by imprisonment or death.[1] Even today, our society does not seem to be able to rest easily with the idea that a significant minority of the population is interested in spending the most intimate moments of their lives with their own gender.

Until the early 1970s, American society had an easy way out on this matter. There had been a long-standing agreement between societal values and psychiatry's understanding that homosexual persons were "sick." The dominant twentieth-century justification for this ancient idea was that heterosexuality was the God-given, natural outcome of biological forces that ensured procreation. Homosexuality was viewed as ungodly, unnatural, unreproductive, and via the medical profession, a consequence of childhood damage—such as traumas, aberrant family processes, or individual problems. Homosexuality was explained as the defensive, easier, and inferior route of loving the same sex rather than risking the anxiety of the higher plane of heterosexual loving. Male homosexuality was thought to be produced by early life factors—most often summarized as overly close, individuation-impeding mothers and indifferent, distant fathers. The explanations of female homosexuality were never as succinctly developed. The sickness of males and females alike, however, was not only a sexual one, but invariably one of character and structure as well.

Today, less than two decades since a panel of experts looked into the scientific merit of the classification of homosexuality as a mental illness and found it wanting, the subject can be discussed more calmly and clearly.[2] What is known can be separated from what is believed. What is believed can be separated into what is supported by data and what is simply a matter of historically reinforced attitudes. Nonetheless, homosexuality remains a profoundly provocative topic.

Since homosexuality is no longer considered an illness, it no longer is an ethically acceptable therapeutic goal to change a person into a heterosexual. The topic of homosexuality is still relevant for clinicians, however. The subject frequently arises in the course of dealing with problems involving gender identity, paraphilia, desire problems, and other sexual dysfunctions. Parents, upon learning their child's homosexual orientation, often will seek out clinicians for some perspective. Distressed teenagers and adults still seek help about their homoeroticism and homosexuality. Homosexual persons have at least the same range of emotional problems that heterosexuals do and may have more substance abuse.[3] And AIDS continues to bring many HIV-infected men to mental health care. Although the mental health professions have formally distanced themselves from the societal values that continue to discriminate against and devalue members of the homosexual subculture, it is important that clinicians understand what is known about homosexuality.

THE DIMENSIONS OF HOMOSEXUALITY

Orientation, like other dimensions of sexual identity, has a subjective and behavioral aspect. The subjective aspect is comprised of private thoughts, fantasies, attractions, dreams, and identity labels that are subsumed under the term *homoeroticism*. The behavioral aspect, subsumed under the term *homosexuality*, involves the objectifiable, more public features, such as partner-seeking behaviors, sexual acts, and political activity as a gay man or lesbian. The subjective and behavioral aspects of this orientation do not invariably correspond. Homosexuality and heterosexuality are not either/or, mutually exclusive phenomena. Many heterosexuals have had some homosexual experiences. Some people are predominantly heterosexual or predominantly homosexual. There are many married women and men who have regular extramarital same-gender sexual experiences. The seven-unit Kinsey scale (see Chapter 3) is often telescoped by saying that a person's orientation is either heterosexual, homosexual, or bisexual (or if eroticism is the focus of measurement, heteroerotic, homoerotic, or bierotic). This summary does not do justice to the diversity among homosexual women and men.

Homosexuality Is Many Things

At the very least, homosexuality is a multidimensional phenomenon involving love, sex, community, and identity. It is a romantic predisposition to emotionally attach and easily love members of the same sex. It is within this context that the more broadly understood erotic and sexual aspects of homosexuality need to be placed by therapists. Homosexuality is also a preference for membership in the subculture of same-sexed homoerotic friends and acquaintances—that is, it is a preference for membership in a community. It is a personal identification with the political issues relevant to that community. Homosexuality is a matter of identity—a label that categorizes the self, clarifies the nature of one's internal and public experiences, and gives meaning to one's life.

Diversity among Homosexual Women and Men

Individuals who share a homosexual identity differ dramatically from one another in their eroticism, sexual experiences, love relationships, relationship to community, and interest in political matters. Bell and Weinberg documented this diversity in their book *The Homosexualities*.[4]

Orientation may be summarized most simply in trichotomous (hetero-, homo-, bi-) terms or appreciated in its love, sex, community, and identity aspects, but its richest reality is seen by adding two additional dimensions to it—evolution and gender.

Evolution of Orientation

Orientation is not fixed permanently in everyone. Homosexual adolescents and young adults often undergo dramatic changes as they decipher and react to their erotic attractions. They may at times label themselves as heterosexual, bisexual, confused, or asexual as they confront the consistency of their most arousing eroticism. Although heterosexuals also undergo adolescent struggles with their eroticism, their conflicts are usually mild when compared with the tasks faced by homosexual teenagers. The need to label and categorize sexual behavior in these terms can create confusion. Although Kinsey and his colleagues labeled a person who had rare homosexual activity as "predominantly heterosexual with incidental homosexuality," few people think of themselves as an incidental homosexual. For many people, sexual behavior just happens and does not require a category; labeling is something that professionals do. Since sexual behaviors are so carefully guarded by privacy, it has been difficult to ever learn the extent of people's sexual involvements.

Researchers have constructed scales to quantify the evolution of homosexual orientation.[5,6] Rating seven or more dimensions of a person's orientation in each of three time phases (past, present, ideal future) is impractical as a clinical tool, however. Nonetheless, psychometric instruments emphasize the idea that homosexual behavior and identity are neither static nor homogeneous phenomena. Relatively little is known about the evolution of orientation as gay men and lesbians age beyond young adulthood.

Variations in Gender Identity and Role

There is an understanding in both gay male and lesbian communities that some of its members display gender role behaviors of the opposite sex and sense themselves either as androgynous or crossed over in their gender identity. Although some of this thinking may be exaggerations for the purpose of mockery of erroneous attitudes that all gay men are feminine and all lesbians are masculine,[7] most of the obvious cross-gender behavioral styles have been present since childhood. In 1973, Saghir and Robbins demonstrated that these cross-gender phenomena are significantly more common in gay male and in lesbian rather than in heterosexual groups.[8] In a contemporary examination of this issue using psychometric measures, homosexual men have been demonstrated to be more feminine and homosexual women to be less feminine than heterosexual control subjects.[9]

POLITICS AND THE CAUSE OF HOMOSEXUALITY

Simply stated and scientifically documented, the cause of homosexuality is not known. Many contrary opinions about this observation exist, however. Sometimes these opinions are fairly stated as beliefs. Frequently, they are posited as well-known facts. Sometimes these "facts" are stated without a hint of awareness of the methodologic complexity involved in ascertaining the answer to the question.

Consider these responses to a hypothetical event. If a gene sequence were discovered to lead to a neural organization that led to strong erotic interest in the same sex, which led to homosexual behavior and identity, some groups would immediately say:

1. This proves that homosexuality is a disorder, a sickness, a mistake of nature!
2. This proves that homosexuality is natural, a normal variant of human development initiated by factors outside of social or psychological experience!

3. We have no interest in the matter because the relevant issues are discrimination, health care, dignity, and developing self-esteem in a hostile environment—not causality.
4. This is of great interest! Here at last are the physiologic underpinnings of what used to be hypothesized as the constitutional contribution to orientation.
5. This is dangerous! The next thing we will hear is that molecular geneticists will be trying to reverse homosexuality through gene therapy.
6. This is great! Maybe the medical scientists will soon find a way to fix homosexuality *in utero*.

This array of responses indicates that progress in delineating the causal influences on homoeroticism and homosexual behavior do not exist in a political vacuum. Data on homosexuality are difficult to examine dispassionately. They are often viewed first in terms of how they may advance or hinder a particular group's interests. These group interests are now beginning to be traced in a scholarly fashion by historians.[10,11]

It is not particularly intellectually satisfying or fair to leave the issue of the causal influences on orientation as "unknown." The field has gone far beyond the simple question, "Is it nature or nurture?"

Variable biological, social, and psychological influences on orientation may account for some of the diversity among homosexual populations.[12] This paradigm leaves room for important interfacing of genetic, prenatal, postnatal, psychological, and social influences. Paradigms are relatively easy, however; evidence that satisfies scientific skepticism is difficult.

Biological Aspects

Periodically the evidence for a biological contribution to orientation is reviewed.[13] This vast literature consists of separate lines of evidence that have been investigated to isolate the proof that a biological push toward a homosexual or bisexual orientation exists. The goal has been to detect the biological conditions under which males and females grow up to be homosexual. Much of the work has proceeded on the assumption that homosexual persons have pseudohermaphroditic brain differentiation—that is, their brains may have an anatomy or physiology that is intermediate between normal male and female forms. Evidence has been sought in multiple areas:

1. Animal models of homosexual behaviors
2. Effect of prenatal hormones on fetal brain development
3. Effect of circulating hormones on adult brain function
4. Estrogen feedback effect on luteinizing hormone (a marker of sex-linked physiology)

5. Differences in size of hypothalamic nuclei between males and females and heterosexual and homosexual males
6. Differences in cerebral cortex between males and females
7. Sex-linked cognitive abilities
8. Behavioral differences between male and female primates
9. Behavioral differences between boys and girls in sex-segregated play
10. Genetic studies of mono- and dizygotic twins and siblings
11. Influence of abnormal prenatal and perinatal endocrine environments associated with: (a) androgen insensitivity syndromes, (b) congenital adrenal hyperplasia, (c) 5-alpha-reductase deficiency, (d) 17-beta-hydroxysteroid dehydrogenase deficiency, (e) exogenous diethylstilbestrol administration to pregnant women, and (f) extreme maternal social stress during pregnancy

In 1990, endocrinologist Gooren and co-workers' review concluded: "It is questionable whether the concept of homosexuality as a form of pseudohermaphroditism of the brain is tenable. That certain (prenatal) biological factors facilitate a homosexual orientation later in life cannot yet be discounted, but irrefutable evidence is presently lacking" (p. 191).[14]

Neuroscientist Hines and research psychiatrist Green's 1991 review concluded, "What emerge currently from the data are perhaps temporary signposts to a multidimensional series of processes that operate at varying interindividual intensities with an equally complex and undetermined constellation of environmental interfaces" (p. 551).[13]

Psychiatrists Friedman and Downey's (personal communication, 1992) review leans tentatively in the direction that biology creates a tendency toward homosexual orientation through prenatal endocrine influences. They place much weight on the fact that most lines of investigation suggest a slight, although inconclusive influence.

No study has ever conclusively demonstrated that a biological factor invariably produces a homosexual or a bisexual orientation. One of the strongest lines of evidence, however, suggests that the excessive androgen exposure that occurs in females with congenital adrenal hyperplasia or adrenogenital syndrome tends to produce more masculine childhood behaviors.[15] This well-documented tomboyish pattern is an intriguing example of the relationship of an abnormal endocrine milieu organizing postnatal gender role behaviors. Preference for masculine behaviors is not the same as homosexuality, however. The vast majority of homosexual persons are normal endocrinologically.

Science is still waiting for the *replicated* missing information that a significant percentage of fetuses containing factor "X" develops a same-sex orientation. In the meantime, there are important lines of investigation of postnatal processes.

WHITHAM'S STUDIES

Although most retrospective research on adults stresses the diverse developmental pathways taken to homosexual orientation, sociologist Whitham's studies on male and female homosexuals in the United States, Brazil, Peru or Guatemala, and the Philippines have shown that childhood behavioral precursors of adult homosexuality are remarkably similar. The precursors of some adult homosexuality are stereotypic cross-gender behavioral play preferences. For example, homosexual men reported patterns of doll play, sewing, cooking, cross-dressing, preferring girl playmates and adult women, and being regarded as a sissy.[16]

Homosexual women reported playing with boys' toys, dressing up as a man rather than as a woman, and being regarded as a tomboy.[17] These societies differed markedly in general cultural conditions, economic development, laws and attitudes toward gay persons, and yet, despite some variations of the parameters measured, the early cross-gender behaviors were remarkably similar. Erotic attraction among some homosexual persons is not the earliest landmark of homosexual orientation; gender role variance is.

Even this powerful link between childhood gender nonconformity and subsequent homosexual orientation does not prove that every gender atypical child develops homosexuality. I suspect that the linkage is far less strong in girls, who generally demonstrate more androgynous play patterns than do boys. The follow-up studies of females with congenital adrenal hyperplasia suggest that the increased incidence of male play patterns was not invariably associated with later homosexuality or bisexuality. Several studies have shown a higher than expected incidence of homosexuality among girls with this condition, but most of these tomboys grow up to be heterosexual.

GREEN'S PROSPECTIVE STUDY OF FEMININE BOYS

In a carefully done, well-matched longitudinal study of feminine and masculine boys who were followed over a decade, Green demonstrated that boyhood effeminacy was an important precursor of adolescent homoeroticism and homosexual behavior.[18] This repeated-measures study confirmed previous clinical follow-up studies which suggested that effeminacy in boys predicted adolescent homosexual identity. This study, like those of Harry,[19] noted that many of the boys lost their femininity as they moved into adolescence. The study began with feminine boys and, therefore, does not illuminate the development pathway from masculine boyhood to homosexual adolescence.

Green's study, *"The Sissy Boy Syndrome" and the Development of Homo-*

sexuality, leaves unanswered the question of the source of the femininity in the subjects. I recommend this study to be read in its entirety because it is an excellent model of the forethought and execution that is required of compelling work in the behavioral sciences.

OTHER HYPOTHESES OF THE CAUSE
OF MALE HOMOSEXUALITY

Because homosexuality is known to all cultures and seems to have a general prevalence between 5% and 10%, the question of cause remains culturally important. During much of this century, psychoanalytic speculations dominated clinical teachings about the cause of homosexuality.

Psychoanalytic Hypotheses

These hypotheses emphasized a constitutional factor plus family dynamics that were partially described in the introduction to this chapter. Family dynamics are understood as including the quality of relationships between members, the effect of these relationship qualities on the child's passage through expected developmental stages, and the internalized aspects of these relationships on the child's images of self, mother, and father. Psychoanalytic ideas have historically been difficult to prove or refute.

When psychoanalytic hypotheses were in ascendance, the concepts of gender identity and gender role behaviors were not formulated, and no prospective studies and few nonpsychoanalytic studies were taken into consideration.[20] Today, although the question of cause is not answered, there is a better awareness of the contrast between the richness that some clinicians find in psychoanalytic work and theory building and its scientific power. The science of psychoanalysis is a retrospective single-case study method that can readily formulate but not actually test hypotheses. Although clinicians and their patients commonly develop a conviction about the cause of unwanted mental phenomena, the scientific establishment of causality is far more complicated.

It is not likely that psychoanalysts will conduct prospective controlled studies of children with close-binding mothers and indifferent fathers to test the hypothesis of Bieber and co-workers about the psychodynamic origin of male homoeroticism. Many studies were done to verify the Bieber conclusions with a moderate degree of confirmation. Eventually, however, researchers began to realize that retrospective findings could not be used to establish causality; for instance, many began to wonder about the role of the child himself in the family dynamics. Seigelman compared the family background of homosexuals to heterosexuals who were low on neuroticism and found that the differences in family interaction patterns disappeared. His conclusion that there probably was not a typical parental background generally present in either most homosexuals or heterosexuals took the power out of the Bieber study.[21]

Friedman's Hypothesis

In an attempt to explain the homosexual men with masculine gender role behavior and identities, Friedman has hypothesized that the persistent sense of unmasculinity during the childhood of masculine-appearing boys may also be a precursor of adolescent homoeroticism.[22] The fact that there are homosexual men who do not recall such juvenile unmasculinity reminds clinicians that gay, identified men are diverse in their developmental backgrounds. In the 25 years between these two psychoanalytic hypotheses, it is apparent that much has been learned about diversity and scientific method.

Sociobiologic Hypothesis

This is not so much a distinct hypothesis as it is an exploration of the possibility that an evolutionary advantage exists for the recurrent appearance of homosexual men and women throughout the ages. Such a hypothesis invites discourse on why "nature" has seen fit to keep generating a type of human being that has distinct reproductive disadvantages.[23] Sociobiological hypotheses of male homosexuality do not preclude the interaction of biological and postnatal influences; they merely try to make sense of the biological forces in terms of advantages for survival of the species.

HYPOTHESES ABOUT THE ORIGINS OF LESBIANISM

The literature concerning the origins of lesbianism is sparse and scientifically limited. The pre-1970s clinical literature, which is almost exclusively psychodynamic, took as an *a priori* assumption that lesbianism was a psychopathology. Case reports concentrated on showing what was wrong with these women. Today, discussions about the developmental processes that lead to a same-sex orientation are unpopular and are almost always suspected of containing the same assumption, that lesbianism is a sickness. The following hypotheses taken together may have some power to explain the diversity of women who develop a lesbian identity.

Outcome of Childhood Gender Role Nonconformity

There has been no follow-up study of masculine girls that is comparable to the prospective studies of feminine boys. Numerous retrospective
controlled studies, however, have shown a strong linkage between childhood nonconformity with feminine gender role behaviors and adult lesbianism. For instance, two-thirds of Saghir and Robins's sample recalled
being tomboys and having wished that they were boys compared to 16%
and 7%, respectively, of heterosexuals. Such studies have led to the hypothesis that some lesbianism is the adolescent and adult orientation outcome of years of childhood cross-gender identification.

Such retrospective data are not as likely to be as correct as the comparable data among males. Female development is probably more complex
than male psychological evolution. It is already known that most tomboys,
for instance, do not become lesbian young adults. The factors that allow for
homosexual and heterosexual development among this group of girls have
not been identified. However, even if the developmental line between
childhood gender role nonconformity and lesbianism is scientifically dis-
cerned in the future, we will be left with the fact that at least one-third
of lesbian-identified women follow a different route to their homosexuality.

There are lesbians who have distinctly masculine behavioral styles,
who value their bodies and enjoy their loving and sexual relationships with
other women as women. These women have been caricatured into the
prototypic lesbian. The perpetuation of this image is a mythic construction
by the culture's collective heterosexual mind.

There is no reason to believe that female psychological development,
even when it is associated with a moderate masculine identification, is
comparable to that of males. Women's greater connectiveness to others,
affiliativeness, and responsiveness to others is obvious from childhood.[24]
These superordinate traits of women apply to most homosexuals as well,
of course, and probably have more influence on their development than
their early-life strong masculine identifications.

This first hypothesis rests heavily on the notion that an early-life af-
finity for cross-gender roles is a predisposing factor to homoeroticism. It
stresses a separate line of development for childhood and adolescent eroticism.

Bisexuality Hypothesis

Twentieth century theorists from Freud on have speculated that bisexuality is a fundamental human characteristic and that socialization
is responsible for the development of either hetero- or homoeroticism.
Bieroticism and bisexuality have rarely been extensively studied or understood. Neither has it been possible to carefully trace the subjective erotic

development of girls. Bieroticism and bisexuality are thought to be significantly more common among females than males.

Speculation arises from these observations that some lesbians are not erotically exclusively homosexual. They may be more aptly described as bisexual. The subjective quality of their psychological and sexual intimacy experiences with each sex leads them to their lesbian identity. This hypothesis emphasizes the impact of identity on erotic orientation. Identification as a lesbian is an emotional, cognitive, and social complexity which is subtly distinct from erotic orientation. This hypothesis may account for some of the women who move from the lesbian community into heterosexual arrangements.

Psychodynamic schools of thought generally assume that orientation is shaped by the balance of internalized objects that a child incorporates as a result of childhood and adolescent experience.[25] The exact mechanisms whereby internalized object relationships shape orientation into bierotic, homoerotic, and heteroerotic molds have not yet been provided.

Pure Homoeroticism Hypothesis

This hypothesis emphasizes that some gender typical girls undergo an erotic development that is consistently homoerotic from late childhood and early adolescence. These girls have a persistent pattern of homoerotic attractions without an erotic interest in males even though their female friends do.

Feminism Ideology Hypothesis

This speculation derives from the powerful changes that occur in some young women as they come to appreciate feminism. They learn about the patriarchal organization of culture. They strongly identify with women and women's issues, and meet, listen to, read about, and interact with lesbian-identified women who teach them about the social and psychological consequences of sexism on women. During this period of rapidly expanding awareness, a sexual experience may help to crystallize a lesbian identity. This hypothesis may account for the fact that some lesbians have been uncomplicated heterosexuals before their epiphany.

TOWARD A THERAPEUTIC ATTITUDE

The heat of the formal debate within the mental health professions about homosexuality has died away, not because of a satisfactory resolution of all the issues, but because arguments over the pathology of homosexuality have lost their fashionability and relevance. AIDS has quickly changed professional priorities concerning homosexuality.

Affirmative Assumptions

Affirmative viewpoints have appeared offering ways for psychotherapists to be helpful to gay men and lesbians. The central feature of this helpfulness is the acceptance of lesbian and gay male orientation as a legitimate and positive guide to identity, loving, and sexual attachment. Affirmative therapy does not assume that heterosexuality is the superior way of life. It is accomplished in different ways by individual therapists.[26] The gay male community approach to affirmative therapy is not identical with that of the lesbian community. For instance, psychotherapy with lesbians often deals with the issues relating to women—for example, sexism, objectification of women's bodies, rape, and incest, whereas the alienation that is highlighted among gay men has more to do with the minority status of their orientation.[27]

Isay has taken some of the same information that psychoanalysts have traditionally used to explain the pathology of homosexual men and has placed a positive view on the natural sequence of unfolding of their orientation.[28] For instance, earlier theorists saw the homosexual man's distant relationship to his father as one of the contributions to his orientation. Isay thinks that the son's sensitivity, artistic interests, gentleness, avoidance of aggressive games, and so forth cause the father's disappointment and withdrawal. He hypothesizes that the son's femininity is an attempt to regain the father's love through imitation of the mother.

Isay has argued that homosexual men can best be helped by accepting the fact that orientation is immutably biologically dictated. He thinks that unfortunate family processes create a variety of sexual problems for gay men, but that homosexual orientation *per se* is not one of them. He views any attempt to cure men of their orientation as dangerous to their self-esteem and recommends that gay men avoid therapists who simply cannot relinquish their cultural biases.

In his scholarly review of the scientific and psychoanalytic literature of male homosexuality, Friedman offered a paradigm to enable therapists to help with the masochism, paranoia, and obsessive-compulsive symptomatology of gay patients without having to interpret their homosexuality as the core of their problems.

Understanding Coming Out

Coming out is a set of complicated developmental tasks unique to lesbian, gay, and bisexual persons that involves psychological recognition and social management of their orientation. The time required, difficulty experienced, and resolution achieved during this elaboration of their identity are highly variable from individual to individual.

Coming out begins with feeling alienated—unlike the heterosexual others in the environment—and alone. Typically this is a prepubertal and early pubertal phase and is triggered by the pressure of recurrent homo-erotic fantasies and attractions. These gradually force the teenager to rec-ognize and label the self as bi- or homosexual. Coming out to the self may be intensely defended against by heterosexual behavior, social isolation, or avoidance of all sexual issues, or may simply lead to homosexual behavior.

Having a consensual same-sex encounter for the first time is usually a profound experience and may contrast dramatically with the subjective lesser pleasure of a previous heterosexual relationship. "I liked that so much, I guess I am gay!" The homosexual experience is an important stim-ulus for self-acceptance. If self-acceptance is enhanced by the experience, select age-mates may then come to be told about one's emerging identity. Increasing social participation in gay male or lesbian groups may ensue. This may be followed by allowing oneself to be known in larger society as a gay person. Many individuals find that the most difficult aspect of coming out is allowing parents to know about their orientation, living arrange-ments, and lover. People take these steps to differing degrees, over varying lengths of time, and with a mixture of positive and negative consequences.

Coming out is emotionally difficult. It forces the person to confront society's derision of homosexuality, to identify the self with a sometimes hated minority, and to face their own internalized derision acquired from being a member of society.

Males generally come out earlier than females in every stage of the process. A study of 270 members of the American Psychological Associa-tion's Task Force on the Status of Lesbian and Gay Male Psychologists, for instance, showed that lesbians recognized their homosexual feelings later and had an intellectual understanding of lesbianism before their first ho-mosexual experience when contrasted to gay men.[29] Their lag between recognition of homoerotic feelings and first homosexual experience was three times longer than for gay men. Lesbians took 10 years to comfortably label themselves as lesbian whereas gay men required 8 years.

Coming out is viewed as a measure of self-respect; it may parallel the internal processes whereby self-esteem is established, affirmed, and re-affirmed. Men and women who are able to be open about their orientation suffer less internally and have more of a sense of personal freedom.

Overcoming Homophobia

Fear or hatred of homosexuality or homosexual persons is referred to as *homophobia*. It can be found throughout the major institutions of our society. Although the governmental, medical, legal, judicial, educational, and other institutions have made progress in recent decades against dis-crimination based on religion, race, age, and sex, almost all institutions are ambivalent about the rights of homosexual persons. Young people in the process of coming out have to be careful that in their zeal to attain personal freedom, they do not underestimate the power of subtle discrimination against them on the basis of their orientation. This is especially true for men in relationship to AIDS.

Homophobia is not simply a matter of negative forces outside the gay person; homophobia is internalized early in life and adds to the burdens of the coming-out process. Therapists working with gay men, lesbians, or bisexual persons should be interested in their patients' coming-out stories; these stories reflect some of their patients' major private struggles. An interest in and understanding of the patient's process of coming out and a willingness to deal with internal and external homophobia offer the patient hope of being helped.

Identification of the Therapist's Orientation

Ordinary mental health institutions, for instance, mental health training clinics in teaching hospitals, initially recognize relatively few gay male and even fewer lesbian patients. Many of these patients are slow to tell the therapist about their orientation, especially when the therapist seems to assume heterosexuality. It is important that therapists act as though they are aware that a significant portion of the population has a homosexual identity.

As homosexual communities become established and better organized, a network of therapists becomes well known to members of the subculture. Homosexual men and women tend to bring their mental health issues to gay-identified therapists or to a few therapists who, although perceived to be heterosexual, are known to lack the usual cultural assumptions about gay people. Gay therapists, especially lesbian therapists, are generally assumed to know firsthand about living with misogyny, homophobia, and the legal barriers against homosexual marriage and child custody. Such therapists feel safer.[30] The gay-identified therapist provides a role model for self-acceptance and community visibility.

This is a departure from how therapist-orientation issues are usually handled in the dominant culture. Generally, therapists are not encouraged to answer patients' questions about their orientation. Rather they are usually instructed to elicit the patient's fantasies and to steer the conversation to the patient's own struggles with orientation. This is what I used to do, but these days, when asked, I reveal my orientation and turn the attention to the patient's reactions.

The Therapeutic Danger

Psychotherapy, the process of helping another person understand the feelings, conflicts, and limitations of the self and to outgrow the constraints that cause suffering, is an art form. It never has successfully been reduced to a technique, a science, or a set of instructions. It usually involves two persons, each of whom has deeply personal relationships to issues relating to gender identity, orientation, the role of women in society, and homophobia.

The management of this relationship is the responsibility of the clinician. Society has left to the therapist the opportunity to work in private, where the words are not heard by others. It is presumed that the issues of the patient, rather than those of the therapist, will hold sway. Insisting that the patient is fundamentally sick because of orientation or that the sickness is due to the unwillingness to come out completely are comparable errors having to do with therapist rather than patient issues.

One safeguard against these countertransference errors is the knowledge that, while the patient expects to learn important things from the educated therapist, the patient is the therapists's teacher. The therapist wants to hear of the struggle, the feelings, and the perspective of the patient. The therapist's perspective is highly valued and powerful but it needs to be understood as ultimately less vital than that of the patient's.

The therapy dialogue is embedded in a relationship that allows for understanding of both the structure of the patient's external and internal worlds. There is always a danger of getting either aspects of the work out of balance. Gay men and lesbian women have other issues to discuss besides their orientation and society's rebuke of it. When a therapist finds that the issues being discussed are only those of orientation, it is time to reconsider whose issues these actually are.

SUMMARY

Homosexual orientation may come about through a series of prepubertal interactive steps that begin with gene-directed protein synthesis, fetal endocrine and brain development, early childhood temperament, family reactions to the child, family processes, gender identity and role evolution, comfort in play activity, and erotic fantasy development. The evolution of orientation does not stop with puberty; it undergoes an even more dramatic and conscious evolution during adolescence. Science has only been able to appreciate these possibilities. In the meantime, homosexual persons have lives to live.

Mental health professionals are occasionally called upon as compassionate, insightful, knowledgable persons to help an individual or a family with their concerns. In order to offer our services without fear, hatred, or misunderstanding, we have to deal privately with our countertransference manifestations of living in a culture that often derides gay males and lesbians as examples of incompetent masculinity and femininity. Qualified clinical services begin with the knowledge that homosexuality is a multidimensional phenomenon involving love, sex, community, and identity; that gay men and lesbians are often psychologically healthy; that the coming-out process is a unique developmental task that creates intense dilemmas for homoerotic adolescents and young adults; and that homosexual persons share an erotic orientation to their own sex although in other identity, sexual function, and nonsexual characteristics they are quite diverse. Homosexual persons are entitled to the best of what our profession has to offer.

REFERENCES

1. Duberman MB, Vicinus M, Chauncecey G: *Hidden from History: Reclaiming the Gay and Lesbian Past.* New York, New American Library, 1989.
2. Bayer R: *Homosexuality and American Psychiatry: The Politics of Diagnosis.* New York, Basic Books, 1981.
3. Cabaj RP: AIDS and chemical dependency: Special issues and treatment barriers for gay and bisexual men. *Journal of Psychoactive Drugs,* 1989; 21(4):387–393.
4. Bell AP, Weinberg MS: *Homosexualities: A Study of Diversity among Men and Women.* New York, Simon & Schuster, 1978.
5. Klein F, Sepekoff B, Wolf TJ: Sexual orientation: A multi-variate dynamic process. *Journal of Homosexuality,* 1985; 11(1/2):35–49.
6. Coleman E: Assessment of sexual orientation. *Journal of Homosexuality,* 1987; 14(1/2):9–24.
7. Isay RA: *Being Homosexual: Gay Men and Their Development.* New York, Farrar, Straus, & Giroux, 1989.
8. Saghir M, Robbins E: *Male and Female Homosexuality.* Baltimore, Williams & Wilkins, 1973.
9. Tuttle GE, Pillard RC: Sexual orientation and cognitive abilities. *Archives of Sexual Behavior,* 1991; 20(3):307–319.
10. Boswell J: *Christianity, Social Tolerance, and Homosexuality.* Chicago, University of Chicago Press, 1980.
11. Greenberg DF: *The Construction of Homosexuality.* Chicago, University of Chicago Press, 1988.
12. Money, J: *Gay, Straight, and In-between.* New York, Oxford University Press, 1988.
13. Hines M, Green R: Human hormonal and neural correlates of sex-typed behaviors, in Tasman A, Goldfinger SM (eds), *Review of Psychiatry, Vol 10,* Washington, American Psychiatric Press, 1991, pp 536–555.
14. Gooren L, Fliers E, Courtney K: Biological determinants of sexual orientation, in Bancroft J (ed), *Annual Review of Sex Research,* Vol I. Lake Mills, Iowa, Society for Scientific Study of Sex, 1990.
15. Dittman RW, Kappes MH, Kappes ME, *et al:* Congenital adrenal hyperplasia II: Gender-related behavior and attitudes in female salt-wasting and simple-viriling patients. *Psychoneuroendocrinology* 1990; 15(5–6): 421–434.
16. Whitham FL, Mathy RM: *Male Homosexuality in Four Societies: Brazil, Guatemala, Philippines, and United States.* New York, Praeger, 1986.
17. Whitham FL, Mathy RM: Childhood cross-gender behavior of homosexual females in Brazil, Peru, the Philippines, and the United States. *Archives of Sexual Behavior,* 1991; 20(2):151–170.
18. Green R: *"Sissy Boy Syndrome" and the Development of Male Homosexuality,* New Haven, Yale University Press, 1987.

19. Harry J: Defeminization and social class. *Archives of Sexual Behavior,* 1985; 14(1):1–12.

20. Bieber I, *et al: Homosexuality: A Psychoanalytic Study of Male Homosexuals.* New York, Basic Books, 1962.

21. Siegelman M: Parental backgrounds of male homosexuals and heterosexuals: A cross-national replication. *Archives of Sexual Behavior,* 1981; 10(6):505–512.

22. Friedman RC: *Male Homosexuality: A Contemporary Psychoanalytic Perspective.* New Haven, Yale University Press. 1988.

23. Weinrich JD: *Sexual Landscapes: Why We Are What We Are, Why We Love Whom We Love.* New York, Charles Scribner's Sons, 1987.

24. Gilligan C: *In a Different Voice: Psychological Theory and Women's Development.* Cambridge, Harvard University Press, 1982.

25. Scharff DE: *The Sexual Relationship: An Object Relations View of the Family.* London, Routledge, Kegan, Paul, 1982.

26. Garnets L, Hancock KA, Cochran SD, *et al:* Issues in psychotherapy with lesbians and gay men. *American Psychologist,* 1991; 46(9):964–972.

27. Falco KL: *Psychotherapy with Lesbian Clients: Theory into Practice.* New York, Brunner/Mazel, 1991.

28. Isay RA: Fathers and their homosexually inclined sons. *Psychoanalytic Study of the Child, Vol 42.* New Haven, Yale University Press, 1987; pp 275–294.

29. Task Force on the Status of Lesbian and Gay Male Psychologists. Removing the stigma. *APA Monitor,* 1977, p 16.

30. Brown, LS: Beyond thou shalt not: Thinking about ethics in the lesbian therapy community. *Women and Therapy,* 1989; 8(1/2):13–25.

CHAPTER 13

Gender Identity Disorders

To the extent that psychopathology illuminates the subtle healthy processes of development, the gender identity disorders teach us about the most fundamental aspects of our sexual selves. Suffering and lost potential abound among the gender-disordered, but so do courage, determination, and triumph of the belief in self-expression.

There is no question about it: there are some people in almost all age groups who rue the day they were born to their biological sex and who long for the opportunity to simply live their lives in a manner befitting the other gender. Clinicians give these children, teenagers, and adults psychiatric diagnoses and thereby designate them as having a mental disorder. But when we get beyond our professional diagnostic paradigm, we see that the most gender-disordered people repudiate the possibility of finding happiness in their culture within the broad framework of roles given to members of their sex by their society.

This repudiation is not primarily motivated by an intellectual attack on sexism, homophobia, or any other injustice embedded in cultural mores. It is motivated by a literal repudiation of the body, of the self in that body, and of performing roles expected of people with that body. It is a subtle, usually self-contained rebellion against society's need to designate them in terms of their biological sex.

The repudiation and rebellion may first occur as a subjective internal drama of fantasy, as behavioral expression in play, or a preference for the company of others. Regardless of when and how it is displayed, the drama of the gender-disordered involves the relentless feeling that "life would be better—easier, fuller, more enjoyable—if I and others could experience me as a member of the opposite sex."

Cross-gender phenomena have been known to exist since early recorded time. The most extreme forms occur infrequently making them easier to label as psychopathology. To the extent that psychopathology refers only to the suffering that follows from irreconcilable conflict and dilemma, people with gender identity disorders clearly have a significant psychopathology. The gender-disordered cannot live their lives as they are without the periodic or constant interfering self-awareness of not being "right."

The drawback to labeling gender identity disorders as psychopathology is that "pathology," when applied to variations of sexual identity, conveys moral reprehensibility or sin. We describe people with depression as having psychopathology without experiencing them as evil, but this is often not so with adolescent and adult gender identity disorders. (Usually, children with gender identity disorders are spared the burden of moral opprobrium.) Clinicians have the responsibility of recognizing and overcoming this tendency to moralize the gender disorders. When moral issues remain in ascendancy, therapists are unable to perceive the nature of the person's underlying developmental problems and are not positioned to grasp how these disorders illuminate the inapparent processes of less extraordinary development.

Tension within the helping professions surfaces quickly when any attempt is made to assist teenagers and adults with profound gender identity disorders. The gender disordered often think they know how to rid themselves of their paralyzing self-consciousness. They have envisioned the solution many times: to live as a member of the opposite gender, to transform their bodies to the extent possible by modern medicine, and to be accepted by all others as the opposite sex. Ultimately, sometimes they are correct; unfortunately, they are not always.

The world in general and the medical world in particular do not quickly come to share this viewpoint. The world, beginning with the family of origin, wants a girl continually to portray herself as a female and wants a boy to portray himself as a male throughout his life. And when a person is unable to conform to this social expectation, society, through its innumerable citizens, labels that person as a freak, weirdo, nut case, evil, dangerous, disturbed, and so forth.

A clinician is called in. The family has one set of hopes, the patient another. The clinician has many tasks, one of which is to mediate between the ambitions of the gender-disordered person and society and see what can be done to help the patient. Unfortunately, countertransference steers most clinicians to deal with their opportunity expeditiously: "Obviously the patient is sick, maybe psychotic, and needs help. I don't take care of people who do these things. Refer *it* out!" With a little supervisory support, however, most clinicians can be helped to be with these human beings. If encouraged to spend a small amount of time with them, therapists soon experience them as possessing some ordinary aspects of their lives and one unusual ambition—they often want to be the opposite sex so badly that they are willing to make it a priority over family, friends, vocation, and material acquisition.

The clinicians who publish guidelines for dealing with the gender-disordered see the extremes of gender impairment. In gender identity clinics, we acquire experience watching patients evolve with cross-gender living, hormone administration, breast and genital surgery. Gender clinics attract patients who seriously consider these dramatic solutions. Everyone who struggles over his or her gender identity and role, however, does not literally wish to make these changes.

Adults who permanently change their bodies to deal with their gender dilemmas represent the far end of the spectrum of adaptations to the problems posed by a significant impairment of gender identity development. Even the lives of the gender-disordered who reject bodily change, however, have been ongoing struggles to come to grips with one developmental task: to develop psychologically and socially in a manner that the family (and the society lurking behind the family, out of the child's view) expects. The intent of this chapter is to focus on gender identity problems without confusing the range of these problems with the well-publicized social, hormonal, and surgical solutions that some people use to deal with them.

THE DIAGNOSIS OF GENDER IDENTITY DISORDER

In nosologic language, a clinician makes the diagnosis of a gender identity disorder when a patient of any age or sex meets these three criteria:[1]

1. A strong and persistent cross-gender identification.
2. A persistent discomfort with one's assigned sex or sense of inappropriateness in that gender role.
3. These two characteristics are not due to a nonpsychiatric condition such as an intersex problem.

Strong Persistent Cross-Gender Identification

Children, especially young ones, may not verbalize enough about their inner experiences to ascertain this criterion with certainty, so the DSM-IV provides the additional guidelines. Children should meet four of the following manifestations of cross-gender identification:

1. A repeatedly stated desire to be, or insistence that he or she is, the opposite sex.
2. In boys, preference for cross-dressing or simulating female attire; in girls, insistence on wearing stereotypical masculine clothing.
3. Strong and persistent preferences for cross-gender roles in fantasy play or persistent fantasies of being the opposite sex.

4. Intense desire to participate in the games and pastimes of the opposite sex.
5. Strong preference for playmates of the opposite sex.

In adolescence and adulthood, this criterion is fulfilled when the patient states the desire to be the opposite sex, frequently passes as the opposite sex, desires to live or be treated as the opposite sex, or has the conviction that his or her feelings and reactions are those typical of the opposite sex.

Persistent Discomfort with One's Assigned Sex or the Sense of Inappropriateness in That Gender Role

This criterion is fulfilled in boys who assert that their penises or testicles are disgusting or will disappear or that it would be better not to have these organs; or who demonstrate an aversion toward rough-and-tumble play and rejection of male stereotypical toys, games, and activities.

In girls, rejection of urinating in a sitting position or the assertion that they do not want to grow breasts or menstruate, or a marked aversion toward normative feminine clothing fulfill this criterion.

Among adolescents and adults, this criterion is fulfilled by the patient's (1) preoccupation with getting rid of one's primary and secondary sex characteristics; (2) thoughts about hormones, surgery, or other physical alterations of the body (electrolysis for beard removal, cricoid cartilage shave to contour the Adam's apple, breast augmentation surgery) to enhance the capacity to pass as a member of the opposite sex; and (3) belief that one was born into the wrong sex.

Not Due to a Nonpsychiatric Medical Condition

This criterion is irrelevant in the vast majority of cases because the patient possesses normal genital anatomy and sexual physiology. When a therapist encounters someone with a gender identity disorder and congenital adrenal hyperplasia, an anomaly of the genitalia, or a chromosomal abnormality, the DSM-IV has instructed clinicians to use the diagnosis Gender Identity Disorder Not Otherwise Specified. An alternative method, however, is to classify the patient as a Gender Identity Disorder and list the physical factor on Axis Three.

Recognized physical abnormalities dating from prenatal processes create nosologic confusion. Unless an etiology of a mental disorder is well established, the DSM-IV aspires to be descriptive rather than etiologic. Although science has been interested in the impact of genetic, chromosomal, endocrine abnormalities on a brain-based predisposition to identify with the opposite gender, most children with a particular abnormality do not develop a gender disorder. Thus, the assumption of etiology may be premature and misleading. The major determinants of gender identity pathology may require an interaction of prenatal and developmental processes rather than being produced directly by the biological defect.

Mental health professionals, unlike epidemiologists, do not generally go out into the community to find people who meet criteria for various disorders. We wait until patients or colleagues request our assistance. It is possible that many children, adolescents, and adults struggle for a while with the gender identity task of development and find an adaptation that does not significantly impair their capacities to function socially, academically, or vocationally. The clinician's view of the gender identity disorders emphasizes significant symptomatology which usually carries with it some impairment of relationship, vocational, and social functioning.

THE DIAGNOSIS OF GENDER IDENTITY DISORDER NOT OTHERWISE SPECIFIED

When specific criteria are rigidly applied during structured evaluations, many patients with a gender problem are seen who do not meet criteria. These patients are diagnosed as having Gender Identity Disorder Not Otherwise Specified. Since this is such a cumbersome label, clinicians often refer to this as GIDNOS—Gender Identity Disorder Not Otherwise Specified. Masculine boys with persistent cross-dressing, isolated adults who want to become a woman shortly after their wives or mothers die, men who want to be rid of their genitals without being feminized, unisexual females who imagine themselves as males but who are terrified of any social expression of their masculine gender identity, masculine lesbians in periodic turmoil over their orientation, and all varieties of unusual clinical presentations should be diagnosed as having GIDNOS.

THE RELATIONSHIP OF GENDER IDENTITY DISORDERS TO ORIENTATION

Almost all sex researchers and clinicians consider the establishment of gender identity in a child to occur prior to the evolution of orientation. Gender identity is the first major psychological aspect of sexuality to form and therefore is the reference point for all subsequent psychological sexual development. Generally, gender identity becomes increasingly apparent between 18 and 36 months of age, during which time the erotic preference for arousal stimulated by one sex is not apparent.

The clarity of distinctions between heterosexual, bisexual, and homosexual orientations rests upon the assumption that the sex and gender of the person and the partner are known. When a person designates herself as a lesbian, it is understood to mean she is erotically attracted to another woman. What meaning does "lesbian" have if the woman says she feels she is a man and then lives as a man? She then says, "I am heterosexual, I think of myself as a man; men are attracted to women as am I!" The baffled clinician may think, "Oh no, you are a female, therefore you are a lesbian!" Identity is a self-label, even though clinicians and researchers sometimes find themselves labeling others. To deal with these perplexing issues of whether to use biological sex or psychological gender identity as a reference point, the DSM-IV suggests that adults with gender identity disorders be simply subgrouped according to which sex the patient is sexually attracted: males, females, both, neither.

This makes sense for most gender patients because it is their gender identity that is most important to them. Some are rigid about the sex they are attracted to because it supports their idea about their gender, others are bierotic and are not too concerned with their orientation, still others have not had enough experiences to overcome their uncertainty about their orientation. A few gender patients find all partners too complicated and are only interested in themselves.

Here is just one example of the unusual juxtapositions possible between gender and orientation among the gender-disordered. A young adult female, who has always been attracted to males, after unsuccessfully trying to find her identity within the homosexual community, now aspires to become a man. She wants to change her sex. Her plans are to live as a gay man. Using the DSM-IV, she would be subtyped as attracted to males.

EXTREMELY FEMININE BOYS

Histories provided by parents of feminine sons occasionally generate anecdotes about feminine interests early in their second year of life. Typically, the femininity of these boys is apparent in many ways by the third year. Within that year and the next, playmate preferences often become apparent. Same-sex playmate preference is a typical characteristic of young children.[2] Cross-gender-identified children consistently demonstrate the opposite preference. This has serious consequences for boys in terms of social rejection and living as loners among peers through much of the school years. Masculine girls, in contrast, are accepted better among other girls. Zucker has demonstrated that the peer problems of feminine boys cause some of their behavioral and emotional problems. This psychopathology is particularly clear by middle-to-late childhood.[3] Clinical impressions and psychometric studies also indicate that feminine boys have emotional problems even before peer relationships become a factor. Coates and Person, for instance, emphasized that young feminine boys are depressed and have difficulties with separation anxiety.[4]

Clinical speculations about the etiology of boyhood femininity generally fit the model of cumulative forces converging to create the problem, rather than one factor generating this unusual childhood pattern. Causal formulations of any child's cross-gender identifications are likely to involve constitutional forces, problematic interactions with parents, problematic internal processing of life experiences, and family misfortune—financial, reproductive, physical disease, emotional illness, or death of vital persons. These are sometimes summarized as temperament, disturbed family functioning, separation-individuation problems, and trauma. Occasionally, they are summarized as "unknown."

In the nuance of early life psychosocial processes, temperament is defined not only as the predisposition to respond to the world in a certain way, but also as the aspects that others respond to in the child. Coates has summarized the temperamental factors that she frequently finds in her work with feminine boys:[5]

1. A sense of body fragility and vulnerability that leads to the avoidance of rough-and-tumble play
2. Timidity and fearfulness in the face of new situations
3. A vulnerability to separation and loss
4. An unusual capacity for positive emotional connection to others
5. An ability to imitate
6. Sensitivities to sound, color, texture, odor, temperature, and pain.*

The development of femininity is speculated to occur within the mind of the toddler in response to a loss of emotional availability of the nurturant parent—typically the mother. The lack of maternal availability can be due to a variety of impairments. Because of constitutional predispositions, the child creates a maternal (feminine) self through imitation and fantasy in order to make up for the mother's temporary emotional unavailability. This occurs beyond the family's awareness and is left in place by the family's either ignoring what has transpired in the son or valuing it.

The process of the establishment of boyhood femininity sometimes appears to the family and researchers to be simply constitutional. Those who favor a postnatal explanation disagree and speculate that femininity occurs adaptively, creatively from the boy himself. The boy's problem is that reality is unyielding on gender issues; the adaptive early solution becomes more maladaptive over time. Boyhood femininity is, in essence, a relatively rare accident of development requiring a number of factors to be

---

*Without labeling it as such, the biology of temperament was discussed in the previous chapter in the section on the biological influences on orientation. It is apparent that there is a large gap between the complex postnatal interactions set up by a temperamental characteristic and the measurement of a biological factor, such as prenatal androgen concentrations, in an attempt to predict a postnatal outcome. The biological approach and the psychosocial approach are not competitive either/or influences; in different ways they are trying to account for the shaping forces on gender identity and orientation.

in place, including emotional difficulties of parents and the child's temperamental vulnerabilities and capacities.

Science is far from completely satisfied with this hypothesis. One of the many points it rests upon is a comparison of psychopathology measures among the families of the gender-disturbed, other disturbed children, and controls. At least one study supports the conclusion that the mothers of feminine boys are more disturbed than controls.[6]

MASCULINE GIRLS: TOMBOYS

The masculinity of girls may become apparent as early as age 2, at the same time femininity in boys becomes apparent. The numbers of girls brought to clinical attention for cross-gendered behaviors, self-statements, and aspirations is consistently less than boys by a factor of 1:5 at any age of childhood. It is not known whether this reflects a genuine difference in incidence of gender disorder, the negative meanings that femininity in boys have in our culture relative to the neutral-to-positive meanings of masculinity in girls, or an intuitive understanding that the condition more accurately predicts homosexuality in boys than in girls.

The distinctions between tomboys and gender-disordered girls may be difficult to make. In general, it is a matter of degree. Tomboys are not thought of as being deeply unhappy about their femaleness, or unable to occasionally dress in stereotypic female clothing, or as having a profound aversion to their current and future pubertal anatomic and physiologic transformations. Tomboys are able to enjoy some stereotypic feminine activities along with their obvious pleasures in toys, games, and the company of boys.

These clinical judgments should not be made without careful attention to the child's other areas of functioning. Although most lesbians have a history of tomboyish behaviors, most tomboys develop a heterosexual orientation. Girls who are diagnosed as gender-disordered generally seem to have a relentless intensity about their preoccupations and an insistence about their future. The onset of their cross-gendered identifications is early in life. When a clinician encounters a girl whose clinical picture is uncertain, it is sufficient to recognize that gender is being developmentally processed, whatever diagnostic label is provided; the patient should be followed.

ADOLESCENT GENDER PROBLEMS

Follow-up studies have demonstrated that feminine boys generally lose much of their overt femininity with age. What begins as a struggle over gender identity and role frequently ends up as a homoerotic/bisexual, bierotic/bisexual, or homoerotic/homosexual orientation. Scientific evidence suggests that this outcome occurs in at least 66% of feminine boys.[7] Gender may or may not be a continuing issue for these boys. The specific processes whereby this evolution occurs—when and how, which factors account for gender resolution or continued struggle with gender—are not yet clear. During early adolescence, concepts of gender and orientation may be opposite sides of the same coin until several more years of development transpire that enable them to be separate components of sexual identity.

Clinicians may be called upon to evaluate and provide help with teenagers whose gender and orientation are of uncertain evolution. The patients may not be able to discuss these aspects of themselves. The therapist is unable to discern whether the gender identity evolution is stalled, is successfully occurring, is fixated on a transsexual solution, or is a tactic to avoid experiencing personal and familial homophobia. Clinicians need to act as though they are aware that this line of development is being dealt with rather than simply placing the person in another diagnostic category, such as antisocial personality, substance abuse, or peptic ulcer.

Transvestic Fetishism

Adults are frequently seen by specialists in gender disorders who provide histories of having had masculine gender role behaviors, adolescent heteroeroticism, intense sexual arousal to female garments, and occasional heterosexual experience. As adults, they now report that their adolescent arousal to female clothing (fetishism) has been replaced by a sense of tranquility when they are cross-dressed. Their adult heterosexual experiences are often enhanced by the wearing of at least one article of female clothing—usually underwear. Transvestic fetishism does not bring them to the specialist; their increasing preoccupation with living as a woman does. Transvestic fetishism is one avenue followed by men to the request for sex reassignment surgery.

When fetishism is seen in a teenage boy, however, the situation is more confusing. The person is reasonably or convincingly masculine, his cache of female clothing has been discovered, he admits that he began cross-dressing before puberty but it dramatically intensified with puberty, and his parents are deeply concerned. Is this the start of a serious "late-onset" gender disorder or the onset of a paraphilia which now manifests fetishism but which later will take many other forms? As with other unanswerable questions, clinical follow-up is wise.

Masculine teenage girls are occasionally brought for clinical attention. Their histories of grade school tomboyism are usually followed by extremely difficult emotional years following menstruation and breast development. Sullenness, depression, withdrawal, somatic symptoms, drug abuse, identity diffusion, and diverse acting-out behaviors may occur. Clinicians should respect their intuition about rebellious teenagers and ask direct questions about their sense of themselves as females, their attitudes toward their bodies, and their aspirations.

A 17-year-old and her mother sought consultation for sex reassignment surgery. Jack had been going to school for 5 years as a boy. The relentless tomboyism of grade school was followed by a stubborn insistence that "I am a boy" and a refusal to participate in any relationships that labeled him a girl. The family complied. The school insisted on psychiatric counseling at age 12, but the child was uncooperative with the doctor and therapy was declared unproductive. Since Jack was well-liked, a straight A student, and masculine in manner, "he" was excused from gym class and participated quietly in school as a male. Generally a quiet person, Jack bound his breasts, always wore a baseball cap, socialized with boys in school, and ogled but never dated girls. He did occasionally participate in the social activities at church as one of the boys. During the seventh grade, Jack was treated for headaches and dyspepsia and had a negative ulcer workup.

ADULTS WITH GENDER IDENTITY DISORDERS

The DSM-IV has done away with the term *transsexualism,* which previously was used as a diagnosis of a type of gender disorder. Several factors influenced this decision: people who were labeled as transsexual had remarkably different gender and orientation developmental backgrounds; many people with symptoms of gender identity problems—gender dysphoria—find adaptations that do not involve sex reassignment surgery; the decision to undergo surgical transformation and live in the aspired-to gender was recognized as one solution to a gender identity disorder rather than a requirement for the diagnosis. This change in nosology has the potential of increasing clinical perceptions of the gender problems that are solved nonsurgically.

Most people who request evaluation in a gender identity clinic are at least temporarily seriously considering sex reassignment surgery. Almost all have a gender identity disorder, a few have a complex paraphilic disorder. The majority of the gender-disordered apparently do not proceed to sex reassignment surgery. For some, because they never are able to afford it; in most of the United States, there is no health insurance coverage for sex reassignment surgery. For others, surgery is just too irrevocable a step; they cross-live without undergoing surgery. A few decide that they will find some other means of dealing with their gender identity problems.

In Canada and in other countries where sex reassignment surgery is covered by the national health insurance system, however, a far greater percentage of those originally evaluated as gender-disordered have surgery.

The adults who request evaluation at gender identity clinics tend to fall into the categories described below.

Biological Males

The Consistently Feminine "Heterosexual" Male

Prior to Green's surprising demonstration that only 1 of 44 feminine boys become transsexual by late adolescence,[8] it was assumed that childhood gender disorder was the first form of transsexualism. Although this is not so, gender clinics see patients who provide a corroborated history of relentless femininity throughout childhood, adolescence, and adulthood. They generally are intensely homophobic people who desire to marry a "normal" man.

The Feminine "Homosexual" Male

Some patients, usually from economically disadvantaged families who have survived on the streets from teenage years on, have spent years on the fringe of the homosexual subculture. They have thought of themselves as drag queens, female impersonators, or gay males* who prefer to live or work part-time as women. Some have survived as prostitutes for gay or heterosexual men. Many have been drug dependent. These patients are initially attracted to men during their adolescence but as they begin to live only as women, they may reconsider themselves as bisexual or heterosexual.

The Cross-Dressing Masculine "Heterosexual" Male

These males are the former fetishistic transvestites whose lives superficially appear to be conventional. They sometimes marry, father children, work at high-level jobs, but cross-dress in privacy, with or without the knowledge of their wives. Although they may report that they have felt unconfident about their masculinity prior to puberty, their play patterns and general behaviors typically did not alert their families to any gender difficulties. Cross-dressing typically began before puberty, but almost always by midadolescence. These men have traditionally been labeled *transvestites*.

Transvestites have been confusing for nosologists, who have not been able to decide to categorize them as primarily gender-disordered, paraphilic, or both. This confusion is well founded. Cross-dressing is associated with

---

*For reasons that are not entirely clear, it has become the convention not to refer to gay men who cross-dress as transvestites, although some of the men refer to themselves in this way.

fantasies and self-images of being a woman, even though the female garments may enhance heterosexual desire and potency. Cross-dressing in apparently heterosexual males presents two dominant patterns, each of which may occasionally lead to the request for sex-reassignment surgery. Both of the following patterns have sometimes been referred to as *gender dysphoric transvestites*.

"Simple" Transvestism. The man's fantasies during masturbation and partner sex suggest that transvestism should be thought of as a gender identity pathology. These typically are: during masturbation, that he is a woman having sex with a man; with a partner, that their bodies are reversed—that is, his penis is viewed as hers entering his vagina. The progress is from adolescent fetishistic transvestism to adult nonfetishistic transvestism to increasing preoccupation with living in a female gender role. These men are only "simple" transvestites in the sense that they do not seem to have multiple or progressive paraphilic preoccupations.

Paraphilic Transvestism. The patterns that lead cross-dressing to be diagnosed as a paraphilia are typically masochism, sadism, autoerotic-asphyxia,[9] and its occurrence among those who commit sex offenses. Perhaps the most well-known form of transvestism through the ages is that associated with bondage, domination by a powerful woman, and sadistic role reversals.

The psychodynamics of such cases are often thought to demonstrate denial of the differences between the sexes, reassurance that women have penises, castration anxiety, and submitting to the traumatic forcefulness of mother in a controlled stylized way in order to master early life humiliations.[10]

Blanchard has recently delineated a small group of men who request sex reassignment surgery who, rather than being attracted to males or females or being aroused by female clothing, are aroused by images of themselves as women. He terms these males *autogynephilics*[11] and considers them asexual in their orientation. Although most men with autogynephilia cross-dress and some pursue sex-reassignment surgery, he has interviewed men with this erotic preoccupation who do not cross-dress; they simply masturbate to images of themselves as women. I am not sure that autogynephils should be thought of as a third pattern of transvestism that occasionally leads to the request for sex-reassignment surgery. Blanchard may have identified the erotic fantasy that is unique to all transvestites, and that men who fall into his category are more inhibited in their expressions of the central fantasy. If autogynephilia cannot be viewed as the most schizoid-narcissistic of the transvestisms, it at least stands as a reminder that the pathologies of sexual identity have many subtle variations, some of which are behavioral and some purely erotic.

Most of the transvestism that clinicians see at gender clinics are men whose need for expression of their female selves can no longer be contained through solitary cross-dressing and occasional social outings as a woman. Sometimes in other settings, however, a transvestite is brought to a therapist by a wife who accidentally has discovered her husband in his female attire. Such a man often demonstrates a "simple" transvestism that is relatively well-integrated into his private life—that is, his life is divided into a usual masculine role and a secret compartmentalized female solitary cross-dressing. The sexual function of such men is often characterized by low motivation to make love with their wives. Sexual frequency and potency may dramatically increase if the woman can tolerate his use of female clothing during lovemaking.

> A middle-aged woman requested help for recurrence of major depression. This, her third episode of depressive immobilization, followed her adult son's discovery of her husband's cache of female clothing and his refusal to work with his business partner–father. Her druggist husband started to drink heavily in response to these family and business pressures.
>
> The woman had adapted to her husband's "unusual sexual pattern" almost three decades ago after she discovered it in the second year of marriage (the precipitant of her first depressive episode).
>
> Throughout his adulthood, her husband was happy to briefly cross-dress about twice a month in private and to attend conventions of a transvestite organization for five days a year where he cross-dressed all day. During times of business stress, parental illness and death, however, he has had fantasies of living full time as a woman and changing his sex. "But I always knew these were just thoughts and I never took them seriously." For most of his marriage he has been able to enjoy intercourse once or twice a month when he can have something silken and feminine nearby. He helped his wife recover by forswearing the cross-dressing, increasing his long-distance bike riding, stopping all alcohol consumption, and attempting to have sex without any female garments. She repeatedly assured him that stopping his cross-dressing was unnecessary and acknowledged that she might miss it a bit—especially because he was more active and interested sexually when he began wearing panty hose. She recovered from her intractable insomnia and other symptoms in three months, and they both attended the transvestite convention together. The son remained aloof.

Biological Females

Females who request evaluation for sex reassignment surgery generally have either been relentless in their masculine behavioral expressions from early life or have lived a unisexual neutral life because of their intense conflict over living as they aspire. They are typically attracted to women only and have been designated as homosexual in orientation by others,[12] although they themselves are usually homophobic. Most have histories consistent with a diagnosis of childhood gender identity disorder.

In their adolescent "heterosexual" relationships, they have kept their breasts and genitals, which offend and embarrass them, off limits to their partners. Some even have masqueraded as a boy, used a dildo with an inexperienced lover, and only disclosed their biological status to their partner shortly before or after marriage.

Some of the middle-aged females have allowed their understanding and accepting partners, who relate to them as men, to stimulate their clitoris to orgasm.

Lesser degrees of gender identity disorders are seen among females. The features are essentially the same, the degree of suffering is less. They may have tried to live as lesbians but their gender identity and their discomfort with their bodies get in the way. If they have tried heterosexual activities, their experiences are often captured by this quote; "I don't feel right being with a man. I'm not interested in his body and I don't like his interest in mine."

TREATMENT OPTIONS FOR ADULTS

The treatment of any gender identity disorder begins after as careful evaluation as possible, including parents, other family members, spouses, psychometric testing, and occasionally physical and laboratory examination. The details will depend on the age of the patient. The recognition of a severe gender identity disorder is usually not difficult. The differential diagnosis is not extensive. The diagnostic conundrums are sometimes caused by questions of the coexistence of low intelligence, organicity, character pathology, paraphilia, and childhood histories of profound physical, emotional, and sexual abuse. It is possible to have a gender identity disorder as well as a psychosis, dysthymia, or other psychiatric diagnosis.

Evaluation

Courage is required for a person to undergo an evaluation for a gender identity problem. About one-half of the people who call our clinic do not complete their evaluation; about one-fourth drop out prior to their first visit. Those who do complete the evaluation often misunderstand what the therapist wants to know. Therapists want to know who they are, what they suffer with, what they have already tried, and how they think and relate. However, the patients often erroneously think they have to prove the purity of their cross-gender identity and past. In the past, this has created the reputation of transsexual patients as unreliable, untrustworthy historians. The problem seems to have improved in recent years after these patients learned that surgery did not require an early-life onset of cross-gender role behaviors.

The evaluation should be a helpful experience for the person with a gender problem. It provides a relationship with a person who is not only interested in their sexual identity but their lives in general. Therapists can answer questions for them, decrease their urgency about starting hormones and having surgery, and help them address the other important issues in their lives. In our gender clinic, the evaluation usually lasts 4 hours extended over several weeks and includes psychometric studies.

Individual Psychotherapy

No one knows how to cure a gender problem. People who have lived long with profound cross-gender identifications do not get insight, behaviorally modified, or medicated and find that they have subsequently a conventional sexual identity. Even with psychoanalysis, 5 days a week for years, the years of living with nonconforming gender images and wishes do not just disappear.

Psychotherapy is useful, nonetheless.[13] If the patient is able to trust a therapist, there can be much to talk about—family relationships are often painful, barriers to relationship intimacy are profound, and work poses many difficult issues. Most important, however, is the fact that the patient has to make a monumental decision: "Should I go through with cross-gender living, hormone therapy, mastectomy, or genital surgery?" The therapist can allow the patient to recognize that downsides to these decisions exist and to recognize and respect their ambivalence. Completion of the gender transformation process usually takes longer than the patient desires. The therapist can come to be regarded as an important source of support during it.

Group Therapy

Group therapy has decided advantages for gender-disordered people.[14] It allows them to know others with gender problems, decreases their social isolation, and finally allows them to be in a group that does not experience their cross-gender aspirations and their past behaviors as weird. Group members can provide helpful suggestions for grooming and passing better. When skillfully handled, the group process can address some of the characterologic problems of individual patients. Many of the patients are narcissistically preoccupied with their gender transitions and have a hard time being supportive. They may initially be competitive or uncaring about the pain of others. The success of these groups depends on the therapists' skills in patient selection and using the group process.

"Real-Life Test"

The guidelines for managing people who are considering sex-reassignment surgery have been spelled out by the Harry Benjamin International

Gender Dysphoria Association.[15] Harry Benjamin, a student of Magnus Hirshfield,* was one of the first physicians to recognize and treat gender problems.[16]

The most important criterion in the guidelines is passing the so-called real-life test. People are said to have passed this test when they still want to proceed with sex-reassignment surgery after dressing at all times as a member of the opposite sex; legally changing their names and their legal documents; functioning full time as a student or as an employee in their new gender role. Time requirements are placed on the real-life test—for instance, 3 months before hormones are administered, 1 year before mastectomy is performed, 2 years before genital surgery is begun. Time requirements vary from clinic to clinic, however. The reason for the real-life test is to give the patient, who created a transsexual solution in fantasy, an opportunity to experience the solution in social reality. Some people realize during this process that it is not the solution for them.

However, gender patients often pass this test and their economic, psychologic, and interpersonal lives are profoundly changed. Economically, females now working as males increase their incomes, whereas males now living as females tend to make less money.[17] In both sexes, however, gender role reorientation is associated with improvement in measures of psychological function.[18] Love relationships improve for biological females when they live as males, whereas improvement in this parameter of adjustment occurs for biological males after vaginoplasty. Family support for people who change their sex varies from hostile rejection, to none, to welcoming. However, isolation from the family of origin or at least some members of the family is by far the most common response.

Hormone Therapy

Gender programs strongly prefer that hormones be administered by endocrinologists who have a working relationship with the gender clinic and have an understanding of the patient's dilemma. Many patients, especially male-to-female ones, will have taken hormones obtained "on the street" prior to their gender evaluation, generally in doses that far exceed what the endocrinologist would prescribe.

Males

The effects that can be expected from administration of estrogen to a biological male are: breast development, testicular atrophy, decreased sex-

---

*Hirshfield was a German physician, one of the original sexologists, who contributed a book on transvestites that sought to describe their histories and to clearly distinguish them from homosexual men, with whom they were routinely confused during the early part of the twentieth century.

ual drive, decreased semen volume and fertility, softening of the skin, fat redistribution in a female pattern, and a decrease in spontaneous erections. Of these changes, modest breast development is often the largest concern to the patient. Hair growth is not usually affected by estrogens. Many patients elect to have electrolysis for facial hair removal. Side effects within recommended doses are generally not a problem, but some patients develop hypertension, hyperglycemia, lipid abnormalities, thrombophlebitis, and hepatic dysfunction.

The most dramatic effect of hormones is on the sense of well-being. Patients report feeling calmer and happier knowing that their bodies are being chemically demasculinized and feminized. The most common preparation of estrogen given to men during their continuing real-life test is ethynyl estradiol (Estinyl) 0.05 mg daily.

Females

The administration of androgen to females quickly results in an increased sexual drive, clitoral tingling and growth, weight gain, and, after several months, amenorrhea and hoarseness. An increase in muscle mass may be apparent if weight training is undertaken simultaneously. Hair growth may be sparse or lush depending on the patient's genetic potential. Frontal baldness may eventually develop. Androgens are typically administered intramuscularly 200–300 mg/monthly. Androgen administration appears fairly safe, although it is prudent to monitor hepatic, lipid, glucose, electrolyte, and thyroid functioning. Most patients are delighted with their bodily changes, although some are disappointed that they remain short, wide-hipped, relatively hairless men with breasts that do not shrink.

Surgical Therapy

Surgical intervention is the last medical step in this dramatic process. It should never occur without a mental health professional's input, even when the patient provides a heart felt convincing set of reasons to bypass the real-life test, hormones, and therapeutic relationship. Surgery is expensive, time-consuming, at times painful, and has frequent complications and disappointments. Patients are better off having their surgery done by those professionals who are experienced in it.

Surgery can be expected to add further improvements in the lives of patients above and beyond that attained through cross-living and hormone administration. A recent British study compared 20 male-to-female transsexuals who were operated upon within 3 months of evaluation with 20 who were treated routinely by having to wait 2 years for surgery.[19] The early-operated group had more social activities with friends and family, were more active in sports, and had more sexual activity than the waiting group. The early-operated group did better vocationally and had improved measures on five of six psychometric scales.

Males

Surgery in males consists of penectomy, orchiectomy, vaginoplasty, and the fashioning of a labia. The procedures used for these processes, especially for the creation of a neovagina, have evolved over the years. Skin grafts are usually used. Postoperatively, the patient must maintain the patency of the neovagina by initially constantly wearing and then, periodically using, a vaginal dilator. Vaginal stenosis or shortening is a complication, especially if postoperative dilatation has not been diligent. This results in limited capacity for penile-vaginal intercourse.[20]

The quest for a female shape that others will no longer mistake for a male body leads many patients to augmentation mammoplasty and some to cricoid cartilage shave. An occasional patient is encountered who is gripped by the pursuit of more extensive surgical transformation involving plastic surgery of the face or vocal cord repositioning. These patients tend to worry the mental health professional, particularly when the patient seems to pass adequately.

Females

The creation of a male-appearing chest through mastectomies and the contouring of the chest wall is relatively simple surgically and requires only a brief hospital stay. Patients are usually immediately delighted with their new-found freedom, but their fantasies of going shirtless are often jarred by the presence of two noticeable horizontal chest scars.

The creation of a neophallus that can erect, contain a functional urethra throughout its length (enabling urination while standing), and that passes as a penis in a locker room has been an impossible surgical challenge for several decades. Recently, the radial forearm skin graft technique has seemed to position most patients for a good chance of success.[21] The surgery involved is the most time-consuming, technically difficult, and expensive of all the sex-reassignment procedures. Erection is made possible by a penile prosthesis. Many female patients consider themselves sex reassigned when they have a hysterectomy, oophorectomy, and mastectomy. They find a partner who understands the situation and supports the idea of living and loving with female genitals.

OTHER GENDER PROBLEMS

Conflicts and distress over any aspect of sexual identity—gender identity, orientation, or intention—carry a burden of shame and a fear of rejection. This burden explains why many patients with these concerns do not immediately tell their mental health professionals what is bothering them. Instead, they may ask for help for symptoms of anxiety, depression, substance abuse, eating disorder, or other psychiatric problems. If the patient is brought by others for help and receives a diagnosis of conduct disorder, psychopathic or other personality disorder or is otherwise difficult to understand, sexual identity issues may be lurking. People diagnosed as borderline personality disorder often have their sexual identity struggles noticed for diagnostic purposes and then forgotten.

Sexual identity issues are easy to overlook. I, who consider myself knowledgeable about the subject, overlooked it for 2 years with one person.

> A friendless, chronically depressed mother of three nearly grown children was referred for sex therapy after she told her psychiatrist of 9 years that she had lost all interest in having sex with her husband. I saw that she had no interest in sex for herself, was in major distress, and did not want to return to her psychiatrist. We agreed to regularly meet. She was on 14 medications. Within a short time, she taught me that she was trying to spend the rest of her life either in a haze or asleep. She had had multiple major psychiatric syndromes, including vaginismus, anorexia-bulimia, recurrent major depression, self-mutilation, chronic aspirin intoxication, and several suicide attempts. She now had lupus erythematosus, a gastric ulcer, which "unfortunately is not stomach cancer," and several self-induced soft tissue and joint deformities. For 2 years, describing her in my mind with a host of diagnoses, watching one florid psychopathology grip her after another, I became content to offer the comfort of our brief weekly meeting and some control over her outrageous medication abuse before IT hit me.
>
> One day, I saw her differently: her frontal scalp hair was almost pulled out in a male balding pattern, she wore the remaining hair short like a man, masculine air force jacket had several rifle and male sport insignias, and her clothes, in which she had never invested, always were the same uniform— man's jeans and a plain sweatshirt. There was not a hint of anything feminine about her. This day I only saw a person uncomfortable with her femaleness. I asked her about her gender identity. This I-never-have-much-to-say person began a period of animation that lasted several months and began to catalyze a modest recovery. During the next 2 years, she was able to decrease her medications to two psychotropic and three other compounds, to come less often, and to report that she was not as depressed. She began to organize several of her days each week with activity. Of course, she talked about hating being a girl, her tomboyishness and her father's positive response to it, her refusal to wear dresses, her misery over her menarche, her hatred of her breasts, her failed attempts to make it as a teenage girl, her marrying an uncomfortable silent man in her twenties, her rush to have babies, her hatred of sexual activity countered only by her wish to do right by him. Raising small children was the only thing in her life that provided her any memorable pleasure.

When this woman began to be a psychiatric patient, psychiatry did not have the language to describe sexual identity. Because I saw so much other psychopathology and experienced her as so hopeless, I was blinded to what was underneath her easily categorizable suffering. Was she borderline, anorectic, addicted, depressed, and sexually dysfunctional? Yes, of course, and more. I now wonder whether if one of her earlier therapists could have recognized her gender problems and given her the language to express her dilemmas; perhaps she would not have had to wait until age 50 to understand herself better.

Every clinician will be able to recognize sexual identity problems when the developmental aspects of gender, orientation, and intention are appreciated. The easy-to-recognize syndromes of gender identity disorders instruct us about what can go wrong during development. Their major value for most mental health clinicians does not lie in the challenge to learn how to manage the severe disorders *per se*. The severe disorders help us to recognize and help those far more common patients who are less conflicted and impaired.

> A slightly effeminate middle-aged man—socially isolated, depressed, greatly overweight, in debt from impulsive shopping—sought help because he became disgusted with himself for cruising the parks for homosexual partners instead of trying to have a relationship. During his fifth psychotherapy session he developed a brief but intense resistance. When he was able to share its content, he prefaced his revelation with, "You will think I am crazy." With much shame, he revealed his recurrent fantasies of being a woman. "I have always wanted to be a girl. I hate myself as I am, I always have. Sometimes I think I should change my sex."

None of this seemed crazy to me.

"Pseudohomosexuality"

Occasionally, clinicians encounter anxious young adult heterosexual men who, after sensing themselves to be serious failures in their male gender roles, develop homoerotic preoccupations. Ovesey and Woods labeled this state of adaptive failure "pseudohomosexuality," and noted that the underlying motivations involved quests for power and dependency.[22] Pseudohomosexual men do not usually behave homosexually; they worry they are becoming homosexual. Pseudohomosexuality is usually a transient interruption of the evolution of heteroeroticism and is understood as the man's derisive reactions to his failures and his need for and wish to be a powerful effective man. When initially described in 1954, psychiatry was not using the concept of gender or homophobia. Today, these anxious, depressed men are understood as expressing their derision about their gender role failures by mobilizing and self-directing their homophobia and misogyny. Ovesey explained their elaboration of homoerotic imagery as: I am a failure → I am not a man → I am castrated → I am a woman → I am homosexual.[23] In whatever language this is explained, the intimate cultural and mental connections between gender identity and orientation and male disdain for women are once again apparent.

SUMMARY

The gender identity disorders are relatively rare, dramatic syndromes of either repudiation of biologically congruent gender role behaviors or the literal attempts to combine masculine and feminine psychological elements within the self. People in the former group come to be known as transsexuals while those in the latter are labeled as varieties of transvestites. They share a problem of self-differentiation that may be due to a combination of pre- and postnatal forces. Their gender identity disturbance may have been socially manifested within the first 3 years of life or delayed for about 10 years until it is manifested in the privacy of the child's thoughts and eroticism. Although many people can successfully adapt to their early-life or early adolescent gender dilemmas, many others experience other psychiatric symptoms that camouflage their underlying problems from unsuspecting mental health professionals. Clinicians need to include a review of a person's line of gender development in their concept of how to take a history so as not to delay a direct approach to their patient's problems.

REFERENCES

1. Bradley SJ, Blanchard R, Coates S, et al: Interim report of the DSM-IV subcommittee on gender identity disorders. *Archives of Sexual Behavior*, 1991; 20(4):333–344.
2. Maccoby EE, Jacklin CN: Gender segregation in childhood. *Advances in Child Development and Behavior*, 1987; 20:239–287.
3. Zucker KJ: Psychosocial and erotic development in cross-gender identified children. *Canadian Journal of Psychiatry*, 1990; 35(6):487–495.
4. Coates S, Person E: Extreme boyhood femininity: Isolated behavior or pervasive disorder? *Journal of the American Academy of Child Psychiatry*, 1985; 24:702–709.
5. Coates S, Friedman RC, Wolfe S: The etiology of boyhood gender identity disorder: A model for integrating temperament, development and psychodynamics. *Psychoanalytic Dialogues*, 1992; 1:481–523.
6. Marantz S, Coates S: Mothers of boys with gender identity disorder: A comparison of matched controls. *Journal of the American Academy of Child and Adolescent Psychiatry*, 1991; 30:310–315.
7. Zucker KJ, Green R: Psychosexual disorders in children and adolescents. *Journal of Child Psychology and Psychiatry*, 1992; 33:107–151.
8. Green R: *"The Sissy Boy Syndrome" and the Development of Homosexuality*. New Haven, Yale University Press, 1987.
9. Blanchard R, Hucker SJ: Age, transvestism, bondage, and concurrent paraphilic activities in 117 fatal cases of autoerotic asphyxia. *British Journal of Psychiatry*, 1991; 159:371–377.

10. Kaplan L: *Female Perversions: The Temptations of Madame Bovary.* New York, Farrar, Straus, Giroux, 1991.
11. Blanchard R: The concept of autogynephilia and the typology of male gender dysphoria. *Journal of Nervous and Mental Diseases,* 1989; 177:616–623.
12. Blanchard R: Gender Identity Disorders in Adult Women, in Blanchard R, Steiner B (eds), *The Clinical Management of Gender Identity Disorders.* Washington, DC, American Psychiatric Press, 1990, pp 79–91.
13. Lothstein LM, Levine SB: Expressive psychotherapy with gender dysphoric patients. *Archives of General Psychiatry* 1981; 38:924–929.
14. Keller AC, Althof SE, Lothstein LM: Group psychotherapy with gender identity patients—a four year study. *American Journal of Psychotherapy,* 1982; 36:223–228.
15. Walker PA, Berger JC, Green R, *et al*: Standards of care: The hormonal and surgical sex reassignment of gender dysphoric persons. *Archives of Sexual Behavior,* 1985; 14:79–90.
16. Benjamin H: *The Transsexual Phenomenon.* New York, Julian Press, 1966.
17. Blanchard R: Gender dysphoria and gender reorientation, in Steiner BW (ed), *Gender Dysphoria: Development, Research, and Management.* New York, Plenum Press. 1985, pp 365–392.
18. Blanchard R, Steiner BW, Clemmensen LH: Gender dysphoria, gender reorientation, and the clinical management of transsexualism. *Journal of Consulting and Clinical Psychology,* 1985; 53:295–304.
19. Mate-Kole C, Freschi M, Robin A: A controlled study of psychological and social change after surgical gender reassignment in selected male transsexuals. *British Journal of Psychiatry,* 1990; 157:261–264.
20. McEwan L, Ceber S, Davis J: Male-to-female surgical genital reassignment, in Walters WAW, Ross MJ (eds), *Transsexualism and Sex Reassignment,* New York, Oxford University Press, 1986.
21. Gilbert DA, Winslow BH, Gilbert DM, *et al*: Transsexual surgery in the genetic female. *Clinics in Plastic Surgery,* 1988; 15(3):471–487.
22. Ovesey L, Woods SM: Pseudohomosexuality and homosexuality in men: Psychodynamics as a guide to treatment, in Marmor J (ed), *Homosexual Behavior: A Modern Reappraisal.* New York, Basic Books, 1980, pp 325–341.
23. Ovesey L: The homosexual conflict: An adaptational analysis. *Psychiatry,* 1954; 17:243–50.

CHAPTER 14

Physical Illness and the Sexual Equilibrium

Serious physical illness sometimes enhances sexual life. Even when it is diminished, however, the most important causes are often psychological.

Life-threatening illness and serious chronic disease have sexual consequences. These consequences affect the patient, the partner, their sexual equilibrium, and sometimes other members of the family as well.

The sexual consequences of illness are not pleasant topics and they are not readily addressed by mental health professionals or other health care providers. The emotional impact of illness is, however, frequently dealt with by mental health professionals, especially those interested in consultation-liaison work. In hospital-based contexts, the focus is usually on the individual's new dependency, self-images, regressed behaviors, and subtle organic cognitive dysfunctions. In ambulatory settings, the focus is usually on the changing roles in the family. Insights about the illness experience have enabled us to understand the new worries, emotions, and conflicts of the ill and their potential to revive earlier life struggles.

Serious illness is a significant personal event, of course. It changes the preoccupations and concerns of the patient, partner, and family, and in doing so, usually diminishes the frequency and quality of sexual function. Sometimes all sexual behavior quickly ends with the diagnosis of serious illness. Less frequently, illness may lead to an enhancement of sexual function.

Illness threatens one of the fundamental tasks of sexual development: to develop and maintain a satisfying sexually active life for as long as the body permits. The specific impact of illness on a person's sexual function depends on the interaction of three general forces:

1. Disease factors, such as severity and specific pathophysiology
2. Personal factors, such as age and previous sexual attitudes

3. Partner factors, such as the meanings the illness have for the spouse and prior satisfaction from sexual activity

These interactions are complex and pose formidable methodologic problems to scientifically characterize.[1] Although it is widely assumed that the usual consequence of these interactions is to dampen sexual expression, it is also suspected that how this occurs is somewhat unique to each person and each sexual equilibrium.[2]

MECHANISMS OF SEXUAL IMPAIRMENT

Sexual function is impaired by six separate mechanisms. Each one may be sufficient to reduce the frequency of sexual activity or its quality. In any particular person's life, more than one of these mechanisms may be simultaneously operating. The more that are in effect, the greater the likelihood that the disease will end the patient's sexual activity.

Pathophysiology of the Disease

Physical diseases interfere with sexual physiology by both well- and poorly characterized mechanisms. Even among the diseases that interfere with sexual life by well-defined processes, however, knowledge of the underlying biochemical and cellular mechanisms is limited. Here are four examples:

1. When kidney disease advances to the point of end-stage renal insufficiency, the chemical milieu of the entire body changes. These metabolic shifts almost inevitably impair and often destroy sexual drive and arousal for both sexes. This probably occurs through several converging mechanisms involving neuropathies, vasculopathies, hypertension, depression, and endocrinopathies.[3] Successful renal transplantation, but not dialysis, often improves sexual drive, intercourse frequency, and sexual satisfaction.[4]

2. Diabetes mellitus frequently produces an autonomic neuropathy of the nervi ergentes proximal to and within the penis. At least 50% of diabetic men at age 50 can no longer depend on their erectile function.[5] Many men with childhood-onset, insulin-dependent Type I diabetes lose their potency several decades earlier than those with Type II diabetes.

3. Spinal cord lesions regardless of whether they are due to trauma, tumor, infection, or multiple sclerosis interfere with neural transmission between the brain and the genitals. Depending on the location and extent of the spinal cord lesions, erection, lubrication, and orgasm problems result.[6]

4. Sjorgren's syndrome, an autoimmune disease, interferes with lac-

rimal, salivary, and vaginal secretions. The dry vagina that results creates dyspareunia.

Many diseases create anatomic and biochemical alterations at many sites in the body and through multiple pathophysiologic mechanisms. Chronic alcoholism, for example, can lead to alteration in the metabolism of androgen and estrogen, create testicular atrophy and brain degeneration, and interfere with peripheral nerve transmission. It is known that alcoholics have more sexual problems, but identifying the specific contribution of endocrine, metabolic, and anatomic factors is usually not possible with certainty. Before some cancers are diagnosed and treated, they may generate metabolic and anatomic disturbances that create both desire problems and genital impairments. Multiple sclerosis, a disease characterized by numerous lesions at many levels of the central nervous system, can interfere with sexual function in several ways.

All serious disease can nonspecifically affect sexual life through fatigue, limitations of energy, and reduced sexual drive. How the latter occurs is still a mystery.

Effects of Surgery

Surgical treatment of some disease processes interrupts the neural coordination of genital function rendering the man or woman sexually dysfunctional. Some of these impairments are relatively minor, such as the retrograde ejaculation that follows the transurethral resection of the prostate for benign prostatic hypertrophy. Other operations—total prostatectomy, colectomy, cystectomy, and aneurysmectomy of the terminal aorta—remove some of the autonomic nerve supply to the genitals. These procedures typically produce an inability to erect; it is less clear how often women's arousal mechanisms are impaired by surgery involving the retroperitoneal space.

Hysterectomy and oophorectomy generally produce no lasting change in sexual function, especially when hormone replacement therapy is provided postoperatively. But these surgeries induce a change in orgasmic patterns for some women and render a small percentage dysfunctional, even after estrogen, progesterone, and androgen are replaced.* Surgery for cancer of the external genitals often removes the labia and clitoris resulting in both negative feelings about appearance and the need to rely on vaginal stimulation for orgasmic attainment.

---

*There is much to learn about the relationship between sexual function, hormonal fluctuations, and function of estrogen and androgen receptors in the brain. Aside from the genital tract, these receptors are found in the pituitary, the preoptic area of the hypothalamus, the amygdala, the hippocampus, and the cortex. Surgical removal of the ovary prior to naturally occurring menopause is a model of a local surgical procedure that induces a metabolic or endocrine change at a distant site—that is, the brain.

Medication Effects

The most common assaults on the biological substrate of sexual function come from medication. When the disease itself is known to lead to sexual dysfunction, the medications are an additional burden on sexual physiology. Untreated hypertensive men, for instance, have a higher prevalence of erectile impairments than do age-matched controls.[7] This suggests that hypertension itself or one of the factors that lead to sustained elevated blood pressure generates erectile dysfunction in some men. When men are treated with one antihypertensive agent, the prevalence of erectile impairment increases. When a second drug is added, the prevalence increases further.[8] The drugs that seem to be particularly harmful are those that impair the sympathetic nervous system through alpha-adrenergic stimulation or beta-adrenergic blockage. Older drugs, such as reserpine and guanethidine, and newer drugs, such as propranolol and clonidine, interfere with arousal mechanisms. Diuretics, especially when used in combination with other antihypertensive agents, are also detrimental to sexual drive and potency.[9]

Commonly used medications may create sexual dysfunction even when the disease itself has no specific impact on sexual function—that is, sexual dysfunction can be a pure side effect. Cimetidine, a potent inhibitor of gastric acid secretion via histamine receptor antagonism, can raise prolactin levels and lead to loss of sexual drive and potency in sexually functional men.[10] Corticosteroids, used for a variety of inflammatory diseases, may cause the woman or man to develop diverse sexual symptoms, including too little or too much sexual drive. A depressed person may develop anorgasmia in response to antidepressants. This has been especially common with the serotonergic drugs, fluoxetine and clomipramine. The anorgasmia and retarded ejaculation are dose related and are readily restored by discontinuing the medication. Women with breast cancer are often given an estrogen receptor blocker, tamoxifen, which can create sexually problematic vaginal dryness. Chemotherapy for various forms of cancer are often treated with combinations of powerful medications that can have profound effects on sexual drive and arousal mechanisms involving the brain, the peripheral nerves, or the genitals. Men who are placed on digitalis for congestive heart failure or arrhythmias may lose their drive and potency in response to the lowered testosterone, increased estradiol, and increased luteinizing hormone (LH) levels.

Radiation

When directed to the pelvis, this cancer therapy causes scarring of the blood vessels, neural damage, and tissue shrinkage that may impair potency or make vaginal intercourse impossible because of vaginal stenosis.

Similarly, when radiation is directed at the spinal cord or brain, tissue damage may interfere with the neurotransmission and create sexual drive, arousal, and orgasm problems.

Patient's Emotional Reactions to Illness

Sexual function is also threatened by the changes that illness brings about in the psychological and social dimensions of a person's life.[11] Serious illness creates new feelings about the self, new challenges to self-esteem, grief about lost capacities, and a new balance of power in the nonsexual relationship. It also presents a series of new adaptive challenges to independence, autonomy, and life-style. Valued activities have to be given up, energy stores become more limited, and time is managed differently. These emotional reactions to these challenges are briefly observable in hospitals and ambulatory settings as the sick begin to appreciate what has happened to them. The adaptive challenges and redefinition of the self as impaired or vulnerable continue long after the patient is medically stabilized, however. When asked about these processes, people often give an anxious laugh and say that the illness has changed so much that the details are too numerous to remember. "Life is just changed!"

Here is a prototypical example of sexual dysfunction resulting from the person's emotional reactions to changes in health.

During the first year after myocardial infarction there is a high incidence of premature ejaculation and erectile problems, even among those on no medications.[12] The cardiac patient's performance anxiety is more complicated than that of physically well men who develop dysfunctions; it operates on two important levels. These men watch themselves during sex to see if they are developing chest pain or shortness of breath. Initially, they are prone to confuse the increase of heart rate and respiration that is part of sexual arousal with cardiac symptoms. This anxious mental focus during sex is sufficient to prevent erection or cause a speedy sex-ending ejaculation. When sexual dysfunction occurs, the ordinary male anxiety over performance is added to the cardiac anxiety. Even when the physician specifically reassures the patient that he may resume sexual intercourse, most men remain anxious. As the anxiety during sexual arousal begins to slowly dissipate during the first several months of less frequent sexual relations, sex may continue to be far less emotionally satisfying for the man.

Partner Reactions to Illness

To continue this cardiac example, the man's anxiety about having angina, arrhythmia, another heart attack, or sudden death during sex explains only half of the sexual anxiety in the bedroom. His partner contributes the rest. Sometimes the partner's anxiety about creating another cardiac event is even greater than the patient's. This depends on whose denial mechanisms are stronger. If both partners use avoidance of sex rather than denial as a means of coping with these worries, the couple may simply not resume sex until each is sure nothing adverse is likely to happen. This can take months or years for some.

When sex does not resume after a serious illness, the clinician needs to consider the degree to which each one of these factors may apply:

1. The patient's feelings about the illness are causing sexual avoidance.
2. The partner's own feelings about the illness are causing sexual avoidance.
3. The partner is avoiding having sex because she intuitively understands his fear and chooses to wait until he can make love with more comfort.
4. The partner is using the illness to avoid sex for reasons that have nothing to do with the illness *per se.*

Sex is conducted within the sexual equilibrium. Each person may provide the motive to avoid resumption of sex. Each person may wish to use the illness as a face-saving device to retreat from the lovemaking arena. Clinicians need to remain alert to the possibility that illness is not the cause of dysfunction, but the solution to long-standing sexual unhappiness.

The resumption of sexual activity after a myocardial infarction offers hope to the man and his partner. The first "normal" sexual experience is often a major symbolic event, standing for the possibility of having a future. Surviving the early sexual experiences unscathed by a repeated cardiac episode or sexual dysfunction not only yields immediate emotional relief, it also is long remembered. For the many patients for whom sexual dysfunction occurs, however, it proves to be another dimension of the new problems induced by the heart disease.

FACTORS THAT IMPEDE SEXUAL RECOVERY FROM PHYSICAL ILLNESS

Most studies of the sexual consequences of physical illness use one-time sampling of subjects to describe the type and extent of sexual problems. These cross-sectional methods produce a range of incidence figures for most disease conditions—for example, the incidence of impotence in the year after a man's first myocardial infarction ranges between 30%–70%. The source of the patients who are studied is crucial to the results since social-economic status correlates with the disease severity, the number of associated diseases, and the other factors that may play a role in producing

sexual dysfunctions. Studies of sexual activity among the physically dis-
eased are improved, of course, by the inclusion of control groups since
even those without illness are known to have a high frequency of sexual
dysfunction. Methodological issues make the scientific basis of knowledge
in this area less compelling than clinical experience. From my experience as
a clinician, the following factors seem to decrease the likelihood of sexual
behavior with a partner after the onset of a serious illness in adulthood.[13]

Increasing Age

Antihypertensive agents produce more impairment in men in their 50s
than in their 40s because the underlying physiological substrate of sexuality is less resilient in each subsequent decade. Similarly, the antiorgasmic
impact of antidepressant medication should be expected to be more powerful in postmenopausal women because their orgasmic capacity is more
tenuous than among younger, regularly orgasmic, menstruating women.

Poor Quality of Sexual Relationship Prior to the Illness

When sex has not been satisfying emotionally, it is far easier to avoid
resuming sexual activity by hiding behind the illness or surgery.[14] The sick
role works well for some people as a means of retiring from sexual activity
well before the body precludes sexual cessation. Prior to illness, sexual
behavior continues because people believe it is normal and important to the
partner despite the fact that the behavior creates anxiety, anger, and disappointment. Even the onset of mild illness may enable a person to withdraw
from sex with a partner.

Poor Quality of Nonsexual Relationship Prior to the Illness

People who are having trouble getting along generally do not have frequent or mutually satisfying sex. Their interpersonal milieu—that is, the ease
the couple has in dealing with the nonsexual demands of life as a couple—and
the quality of reliability and trustworthiness that each has for the other, may
determine the degree of motivation that each partner is able to muster and
sustain when faced with the onset of chronic or life-threatening illness.

Lack of a Partner

A single middle-aged woman who is successfully treated for cancer of
the breast faces several burdens related to her mastectomy that are different from a woman with a partner. "Should I even bother to date?" "When
should I tell him about my surgery?" "How will he react to seeing my

scars?" A single middle-aged man whose second episode of temporary double vision has recently been diagnosed as multiple sclerosis faces issues that other divorced men do not. "Shall I tell her about the diagnosis?" "When?" "Can I believe her when she says that it does not matter?"

Physical disease carries with it a greater uncertainty about the near future than does good physical health. It does matter to partners, even though partners have different ways of minimizing the painful reality. There is a strong tendency to avoid the ill. Partnerless people who are recently seriously ill ask themselves the question, "Who would want me, now?" Elderly widows and widowers whose sexual life is masturbatory with an occasional partner experience tend to conceive of themselves as too old for sexual relations now that they have been treated for cancer or heart disease.

Illness affects self-esteem which in turn affects how people form relationships. This is not to say there is no hope. It is just that there is a new barrier to overcome. Illness also has the potential to open the person's eyes to how others feel about being handicapped. It may dramatically change the attitudes and interests of the person with the illness. People become active in organizations that offer help for those similarly afflicted and may meet new people who provide role models for successful coping with chronic illness.

Medical Severity

The more severe the illness, with continuing functional impairment, the more difficult it will be for the patient and the partner to resume sexual activity. A point is reached in everyone's mental life where the illness precludes the sense of suitability for sex. Individuals with progressive illnesses such as early Alzheimer's disease or metastatic cancer may want to continue to have sex for the partner's sake despite continual symptoms. The husband does this for his wife's self-esteem and his sexual needs. Eventually, however, her cognitive impairment or systemic deterioration ends his willingness to be sexual with her.

> A couple who thought of themselves as fortunate to have been happily married with a wonderful sexual relationship was struck by tragedy. In his middle-forties, the husband developed an inoperable brain tumor. Near death, he awakened at home from a 3-day period of obtundation. His wife was so happy about this apparent respite from what had been an inexorable deterioration that her joy filled him with brief pleasure. During their tearful exchange, he developed an erection. They had their first intercourse in 3 months. He died 4 days later.

In a study of cystic fibrosis, a childhood chronic illness that limits life span to early middle-life, patients showed a variable sexual adjustment depending on personal, spousal, and familial factors. But after a certain level of severe respiratory impairment, no one—male or female—had the energy for or interest in sex.[15]

Poor Disease Acceptance

Illness forces people to grudgingly integrate their unwelcome new reality. Emotions are felt, meanings are processed, and eventually most develop a new identity as a person with the illness—for example, "I am a diabetic." Health professionals recognize poor disease acceptance as a denial of the illness. Denial and poor disease acceptance take many forms— poor medication compliance among adult diabetics, daredevil behavior among teenage boys with hemophilia, unwillingness to make love because of the ostomy bag on the abdomen, unwillingness to use a hearing aid, or refusal to seek medical attention after testing positive for HIV. Another less commonly appreciated aspect of poor disease acceptance is to regard life as holding no further possibilities—that is, denying that an illness can be successfully dealt with.

> A middle-aged truck driver retired because of double vision due to multiple sclerosis. He felt his life to be over. An inarticulate man whose wife had worked, run the house, and raised the children, he was quietly, inactively, and unsuccessfully searching for a way to spend the first two months of his forced retirement, when he developed dizziness and more fatigue. Thereafter, he was sure nothing was possible for him, and he began to avoid the domestic tasks that he had recently undertaken to slightly lighten his wife's burdens. Her chronic resentment toward him then exploded. Between their new arguments in which he claimed sickness and she claimed manipulation, they occasionally tried to make love. His erections were not reliable when with her, although they were more adequate for masturbation and on some mornings. He began to avoid lovemaking, even when his wife said she needed to feel close to him and it did not matter to her if they did not have intercourse. "I can't tolerate the disgrace of my impotence" became a more powerful motivator than the wish to please his wife. She, however, saw in this pattern a further self-centered uncaring response that only infuriated her more. They sought help hoping that his passivity and withdrawal from life were due to depression.

The sexual fate of a couple bearing a chronic illness still rests heavily on the balance of regard for each person's characteristics. Fresh psychogenic sexual problems can be created by new attitudes toward the self and the partner that appear in response to the illness. Hostile, negative, disapproving attitudes can create personal and interpersonal turmoil that ends sexual life, even when the body of the impaired person is still actually able to function sexually.

Concurrent Alcoholism and Substance Abuse

Persons who are addicted to substances and abuse have a handy defense mechanism at their disposal. They can temporarily obliterate their awareness of their emotional pain and leave the responsibility for whatever has to be done to others. Although alcoholism, for example, holds many pathophysiological mysteries about its endocrine, neurologic, metabolic, and psychologic mechanisms, there is little doubt that chronic alcoholism is associated with a much higher prevalence of desire and arousal problems.[16] When substance-abusing people develop an additional serious illness, their coping capacities should not be expected to be high. They are not immune to any of the personal, partner, or sexual equilibrium forces described above; they probably just have less psychological capacity to deal with them.

IMPACT ON THE FAMILY

Little systematic study of the effects of serious illness on the sexual life of other family members has been done. Most information is anecdotal. However, clinicians have opportunities to notice that certain patterns recur. Here are a few:

1. A child is seriously ill. Sexual life between the parents ends because one or both are too preoccupied with worry or too exhausted to make the effort. This can be a dangerous circumstance if one person feels that the spouse is using the health crisis to retire from sexual activity. This is not the inevitable outcome of coping with serious disease in the family. Other couples are able to comfort and support each other with sexual behavior during their frightening, emotionally agonizing time.

2. A mother of school-age children and young adolescents becomes permanently disabled. Progressive deterioration of diseases—such as multiple sclerosis, chronic fatigue syndrome, and amyotrophic lateral sclerosis—change the responsibilities and emotional burdens of each member in a family. In some families, especially those without a strong life-long bond between an alcohol-dependent father and a teenage daughter, there can be a palpable temptation toward incest, which can be played out either by the development of an inordinate closeness between the father and the daughter or actual sexual behavior.

3. A husband becomes disabled. Deprived of sexual and affectionate needs, the wife may eventually become involved with another sexual partner. As the teenage boys become aware of the "disloyalty" and "infidelity" of their mother, they may act out their confusion and conflict by angry sexual behaviors during dating which victimize their sexual partners and eventually add to the burdens of the family.

4. The mother of a teenage girl is diagnosed with metastatic breast cancer. As the family comes to realize the seriousness of the mother's condition, there is so much emotional confusion that the subjective aspects of the children's emotional development often is temporarily lost in the process. The ordinary worries of teenage girls about their own breast development are augmented by what is happening to the mother. Usually the mother is so preoccupied with herself and the more tangible aspects of mothering that the teenager feels emotionally abandoned. This loss of her mother, well before her actual death, may push her prematurely to sexual liaisons in an attempt to comfort and reassure herself that she is intact and that someone is still there for her.

CLINICAL WORK WITH THE CHRONICALLY ILL

Attempts to help the chronically ill to improve their sexual lives can proceed with the knowledge that there are multiple interacting factors at work in every partnerless patient and every couple. The clinician can reasonably begin by asking about the current sexual situation, but if the therapist focuses instead on the quality of sexual experience before the onset of the disease, the present situation will almost always spontaneously emerge. A list of pathogenic influences should be forming in the therapist's mind during the clinical interviews; it should include hypotheses about the organic contributions and psychological ones from the patient and the partner.

In working with the patient or a couple, the therapist can freely acknowledge the complexity of the situation. The therapist should not be misled by patients' remarks that they would like the problem to be a simple one requiring a mere reduction in dosage, the prescription of a vibrator, or being told about a new intercourse technique. These men and women know about their pre-illness problems and their reactions to their life changes in themselves and their partners. They are assured when the therapist's view is not simplistic.

> A 57-year-old woman with several major depressions, chronic dysthymia, and marriage-long complaints about her husband's annoying perfectionism and disapproval of her urged him to seek help for his recurrent impotence. Seven years older, and in robust health, his symptom rapidly improved with a brief couple's therapy. Each partner had a chance to tell what their marriage was like, to articulate their anger, and to affirm their loving commitment to one another. They returned in less than a year because the wife was beginning to develop a chronic pain syndrome that has proven relentless over a decade. During this time, they have been seen monthly supportively and have had periods of adequate intercourse, unilateral lack of desire, and mutual lack of desire. These symptoms bear some relationship to

the sad irony of their lives: their "golden years" are filled with relentless physical pain and emotional despair brought about by the wife's untreatable facial pain.

During this decade, the husband's tendency to psychogenic impotence has been complicated by carcinoma of the prostate which was treated with radiation therapy. This treatment created a distinct loss of penile sensations and erectile firmness. Although mechanically helped by a vacuum device, he could not overcome his humiliation about having to use it. "Anyway, it is no great shakes to have intercourse if you can't feel your penis in the vagina." They have struggled to remain sexually active and can occasionally have intercourse when she has had a good day and when he has not felt angered at her depressive withdrawal. When they do have some sexual contact, both feel better about their lives. Over time, however, sexual behavior has become less frequent and emotionally satisfying as their mutual pain, depression, and desperation have worsened.

Most clinical situations are less complicated because the clinician's involvement with the person or couple is less extensive. Many clinical interventions revolve around one central idea. Here is a vignette involving one of the many demands for accommodation brought about by chronic disease. I learned about it after this aspect was resolved.

A financially successful married father of two daughters has been a model for the good psychosocial outcome possible with hemophilia. His life recently changed with the discovery of his HIV-positive status. He followed his physician's recommendation to take AZT even though he felt fine, seeing the medication as "a ticket to extending the good life." He initially refused to use a condom after his wife was tested and found to be HIV negative. "It is just too much! I can't even be a man the way I want to be anymore. Anyway, you're HIV negative and I'm on AZT, what's the big deal?" His wife, an usually well-informed person about AIDS, told him in no uncertain terms that the big deal was her health, her life, being around to raise their children in case he was not. She became deeply resentful at his cavalier attitude about her health. Three weeks later, he apologized and they resumed their previous regular sexual relationship—with condoms. They then set out to learn about innovative ways to practice safer sex.

Working with the chronically ill is different than working with the physically well in two major ways. First, severe limitations on sexual potential are often imposed by organic factors. Second, the therapist has to face countertransference reactions that reflect awareness that life ends and is often not pleasant while it is ending.

Work with the chronically ill has the same goal as with the non-organically impaired: to help the person or the couple have a sexual life as long as it is physically possible. The experience is varied because serious disease affects children, teenagers, young adults, and others. Almost everyone appreciates the effort to help them find a way of enjoying the same body that has let them down in other ways.

A diagnosis of breast cancer, radical mastectomy, breast reconstruction, and chemotherapy consumed four months of a middle-aged couple's life. Previous to this, their children's problems, his workaholism, and her sense of inadequacy as a mother played major roles in their infrequent sexual contacts and his worry about inadequate erections. They had each seriously considered divorce by the time their last child went away to college. The cancer, however, changed much of their lives for the better. For six years, she has been well, active in helping others who have undergone mastectomies, and has continued to appreciate his constant attentiveness during her chemotherapy. The prospect of confronting death helped each of them reaffirm the importance of their relationship. The fighting decreased noticeably and the children began to comment that it was nicer coming home for vacations. Within six months of the diagnosis, the frequency of their sexual activity increased as did his potency and the ease with which she attained orgasm during intercourse. "I know it sounds funny to say, but I am kind of glad that I had breast cancer because I think we would have divorced without it and now we are much happier together."

SUMMARY

Chronic or life-threatening illness typically accelerates the death of sexual equilibrium. The deterioration of sexual function occurs through varying combinations of biological, psychological, and interpersonal mechanisms. Clinicians may be helpful in restoring or improving sexual function by acknowledging to themselves and their patients that the forces that create the sexual problems are complex and interactive. This prevents simplistic suggestions that only indicate to the patient that the therapist does not grasp the problem.

Scientific study of this area is limited because it is difficult to control the many variables that are clinically thought to shape sexual behavior. It appears, however, that there is considerable individual variation in outcome accounted for by factors that are currently beyond science to measure.

REFERENCES

1. Schover LR, Jensen SB: *Sexuality and Chronic Disease: A Comprehensive Approach.* New York, Guilford Press, 1988.
2. Curry SL, Levine SB, Jones P, Kurit D: Prediction of sexual outcome among women with systemic lupus erythematosus. *Arthritis Care and Research,* 1993; 61(3).
3. Menchini-Fabris GF, Turchi P, Giogi PM, Canale, D: Diagnosis and treatment of sexual dysfunction in patients affected by chronic renal failure on hemodialysis. *Contributions to Nephrology,* 1990; 77:24–33.
4. Muthny FA, Koch U: Quality of life of patients with end-stage renal failure: A comparison

of hemodialysis, CAPD, and transplantation. *Contributions to Nephrology*, 1991; 89:265–273.

5. Rubin A, Babbot D: Impotence and diabetes mellitus. *Journal of the American Medical Association*, 1958; 168:498.

6. Sha'ked, A. (ed.): *Human Sexuality and Rehabilitation Medicine: Sexual Functioning Following Spinal Cord Injury*. Baltimore, Williams & Wilkins, 1981.

7. Bauer GE, Hunyor SN, Baker J, Marshall P: Clinical side effects during antihypertensive treatment: A placebo-controlled double blind study. *Postgraduate Medical Communications*, 1981; 1:49–54.

8. Croog SH, Levine S, Sudilovsky A, *et al*: Sexual symptoms in hypertensive patients: A clinical trial of antihypertensive medications. *Archives of Internal Medicine*, 1988; 148:788–794.

9. Rosen R: Alcohol and drug effects on sexual response: Human experimental and clinical studies, in Bancroft J, Davis CM, Ruppel HJ (eds), *Annual Review of Sex Research: An Integrative and Interdisciplinary Review Vol II*. Lake Mills, Iowa, Society for the Scientific Study of Sex, 1991, pp 119–180.

10. Cantu TG, Korek JS: Central nervous system reactions to histamine 2 receptor blockers. *Annals of Internal Medicine*, 1991, 114:1027–1034.

11. Anderson BL, Jochimsen PR: Sexual functioning among breast cancer, gynecologic cancer, and healthy women. *Journal of Consulting Clinical Psychology*, 1985; 53:25–32.

12. Sjogren K, Fugl-Meyer AR: Some factors influencing quality of life after myocardial infarction. *International Rehabilitation Medicine*, 1983; 5:197–201.

13. Wise TN: Sexual dysfunction in the medically ill. *Psychosomatics*, 1983; 24:787–805.

14. Althof SE, Coffman CB, Levine SB: The effects of coronary bypass surgery on female sexual, psychological, and vocational adaptation. *Journal of Sexual Marital Therapy*, 1984; 10:176–184.

15. Coffman CB, Levine, SB, Althof SE, Stern RC: Sexual adaptation among young adults with cystic fibrosis. *Chest*, 1984; 86:412–418.

16. Schiavi RC: Chronic alcoholism and male sexual dysfunction. *Journal of Sexual and Marital Therapy*, 1990; 16(1):23–33.

CHAPTER 15

Erotic Feelings in Therapy

Part of the fullness of the patient's love is its imagery of the therapist as sexual partner. Why should the patient not love a therapist who consistently provides a high quality affective connection, calm clear thinking, and a reliable interest in the patient's happiness?

The subject of erotic feelings in therapy is difficult for both trainees and practicing therapists. Most of the reasons for this difficulty involve privacy. Although the confidentiality of the therapist–patient relationship is regularly breached in supervision, the subject of a particular patient's erotic transference is burdensome to share whether it is during individual supervision, teaching conferences, or grand rounds. Erotic feelings about a therapist seem undiscussible to therapists for one or more of these reasons: the patient's feelings are difficult to describe in detail; the therapist is usually the last person in the office to become aware of the range and intensity of the patient's feelings; the patient's longings are intensely private and worthy of protection; we worry that we are mishandling the relationship in some way either by causing the intense feelings or not dealing with them appropriately.*

Erotic feelings are usually individually experienced by the patient and therapist within their respective privacies. Patients are often embarrassed by their "irrational" love for their therapists and may initially be appalled at their fantasies of physical intimacies. They have a strong tendency to withhold the topic from discussion. Therapists, particularly those who are just beginning, fear that their erotic responses to their patients are morally reprehensible and perhaps indicate their unsuitability for the role of psychotherapist. When erotic feelings are professionally discussed in supervi-

---

*No less a therapist than Sigmund Freud, when first considering the problem of the patient's love for the doctor, thought that it was provoked by the doctor's failing rather than the situation of therapy. In a letter to his wife concerning Anna O's hysterical childbirth after Breuer abruptly terminated therapy upon learning of her love for him, Freud wrote, "for that to happen one has to be a Breuer." He was to change his mind in a few years.

sion or conferences, the focus is typically on the patient's reactions not the therapist's; supervisors often think that the therapist's erotic responses exist beyond the boundary of supervision. As a result, most therapist–supervisor dyads never deal with the subject.

EROTIC TRANSFERENCES

Of course, the erotic transference is not a new topic to the mental health professions. It has been repeatedly dealt with throughout the history of psychoanalysis beginning with Freud and Breuer's early work before the turn of the century.[1] At various times it has been regarded and understood as a defense, a resistance, and a form of remembering. It has also been viewed as neurotic, psychotic, inappropriate, and essential, a harbinger of a therapeutic stalemate, and an invitation for disaster. More relevant, however, is the fact that the understanding of erotic transferences varies from case to case and from time to time within the same therapeutic relationship. Erotic transferences are not static phenomena that yield to facile interpretations.

The general public understands that it is not unusual for heterosexual women to temporarily fall in love with their male therapists. This female–male dyad, however, is not the only combination of human beings that provokes love and erotic responses within therapeutic settings. Heterosexual men fall in love with their women therapists. Same-sexed dyads of women or men also generate loving and erotic feelings. Two often overlooked factors—the patient's orientation and the quality of the patient's love life—probably play a large role in determining whether the erotic transferences surface early and intensely and are recognized by the therapist.

Orientation

Most heterosexual women do not expect to have erotic feelings for their women therapists; neither do most heterosexual men expect this type of subjective experience about their male therapists. Freedom from the erotic transferences is one of the reasons that men and women seek therapists of their same sex. Some therapies are satisfactorily completed without the therapists' having to give this topic any thought.

Orientation determines vulnerability to falling in love and thinking about people in erotic terms. When both the patient and the therapist are heterosexual and the same sex, each has strong defenses against experiencing the other as erotic objects. This does not mean that erotic transferences will not occur; it does mean, however, that the patient and the therapist may not quickly recognize them.

Quality of the Patient's Love Relationship

Love is a frequently discussed subject in psychodynamic therapies. A loving, requited relationship provides an outlet for sexual excitements that arise within therapy, sometimes beyond the patient's full awareness. Many people seek therapy for problems that relate to their unhappy relationships or the absence of a peer to love. The therapist quickly becomes seen as the person to love. At first, this may seem ridiculous to the therapist who may be decades older or younger than the patient, but hunger to love and be loved is what is contained within the person and given voice in the therapy.

> When I was 35 years old, a woman 35 years my senior, who had been seeing me for support during her beloved husband's inexorable decline with Alzheimer's disease, became annoyed with me because I had never brought up the subject of her current sexuality. "I am not too old to love, you know, and we have been meeting for over a year!" We went on to discuss her previous sexual life, her current masturbation, and her mixed feelings about me as a son and a "man."

Erotic feelings occur to some extent in most lasting therapeutic relationships because they are a product of emotional attachment that arises out of the high quality of psychological intimacy that therapists provide. Although therapists can describe the defensive, resistive, acting out, or other unconscious aspects of this phenomenon, erotic and loving feelings are legitimate psychic realities of the present. This fact is particularly difficult for therapists to assimulate comfortably.

Therapeutic Defensiveness

There is an element of defensiveness on the part of therapists about erotic transferences. We are understandably uncomfortable with the patient's erotic, loving preoccupations, particularly when they are experienced by us as relentless, demanding, or otherwise aggressive (this is sometimes referred to as the *eroticized transference*[2]). We prefer to analyze the patient's emotional intensities as related to earlier important relationships (here we are correct) in the hope that this will relieve us and the patient of its burdens (here we are often not correct).

Why the Therapist Is Loved

The patient subjectively loves the therapist and part of the fullness of this love is its imagery of the therapist as sexual partner. The reasons for this love are not difficult to grasp. From the patient's vantage point, the therapist is the vital ingredient in the relationship. The therapist is devoted to the patient's psychological improvement and skillfully facilitates increasing trust, revelation, and self understanding. The patient's time with the therapist is also valued because their affective connection remains remarkably good over time. The therapist is steady, reliable, interested, curious, calm, warm, understanding, and provides a high quality of psychological intimacy (see Chapter 4). Discussions with the therapist often help the patient think through and come to decisions that have been difficult to make. The patient is grateful.

In the process of experiencing the therapist's personality traits and therapeutic style, the patient often becomes increasingly aware of hidden aspects of the self—for example, anger at family members, contradictory wishes, personal paradoxes, influences of forgotten experiences. Learning about and accepting these aspects is accompanied by many negative and positive affects about the therapist. Over time, these affects may come to be thought of as "love."

The Therapist's Acceptance of the Patient's Love

The therapist tends to think of such love as "transference." This label carries with it an intellectual framework for understanding and analyzing the love. However, the patient thinks the therapist is crazy: "This is real. It is what I feel about you—now!" Often this state of being at loggerheads between the patient and the therapist proves to be a prolonged stalemate. While each has a viewpoint about how to view this love, both are correct and both are defensive about the topic.

When a therapist can accept a person's loving and erotic feelings without fear, the therapist may be allowed to see the extent of the patient's love. This process of talking about loving feelings and fantasies enables the patient to understand that he or she loves in a characteristic way, a way that has been shaped by previous experiences. It also helps the person to become acquainted with his or her own personal admixture of love, fear, defensiveness, and aggression that initially seemed to be pure love for the therapist. This process leaves the patient with a new psychological sophistication.

The work of psychotherapy does not make the love for the therapist go away; it deepens it, tempers it, yields a newer understanding of the growth-promoting aspects of high quality relationships, and helps the patient to see that other people must be equally complex.

Unfortunately, some people leave therapy because of the intensity of the love, the therapist's refusal to gratify the physical demands inherent in the love, and the frustration of being so close to a beloved person who maintains the boundaries of therapy. This accounts for the reputation of erotic transferences as being a sign of a stalemate or therapeutic intractability.[3]

EROTIC COUNTERTRANSFERENCES

The calm, fearless acceptance of the patient's love is not easy to accomplish initially, particularly for those clinicians who are having their first such experience in therapy. First or one-hundredth experience, however, intense personally directed love, presented with an imagery that is designed to arouse and seduce, stirs most therapists—narcissistically, erotically, and intellectually. It is our intellect that we share with the patient. We are paid for our ability to deal with our temptations, fantasies, and arousal with apparent calm. If a videotape of the "calm" therapist's face were available, I feel certain that all could see that "calm" is a relative term. Blushing, swallowing, coughing, shifting in the chair, or slight facial twitches would be apparent. Our sentences probably lose some of their crispness at these times. Human beings, including therapists, are moved by ardent love; we often do not know what to say.

Such intensity is not an everyday experience for the therapist, but the therapist needs to make certain that he or she is not defensively preventing the surfacing of what is the genuine emotional state of the patient.

The Therapist's Erotic Attachment to the Patient

The therapist may come to love the patient in his or her own way, although it is different from the way that the patient loves the therapist. The special environment between clinician and patient is difficult to find outside of therapy. The patient teaches the therapist and the therapist is grateful for the continuing trust and revelation. They are a team. The therapist's affection, pleasure, and gratitude—love—periodically have erotic representation.

Some of these erotic responses may be a reflection of what is unsaid between the patient and the therapist. The attunement of the therapist to the patient may be such that the patient's unspoken erotic preoccupation with the therapist creates an erotic response in the therapist even though the language that is passing between them does not indicate any such preoccupation.[4]

> All I noticed at first was that she was dressing in a fancier fashion than my other patients. Her clothing had a lacy, elaborate, old-worldly feminine feel. She looked lovely in her carefully prepared way, but there was something sad about this. I initially thought her overdressing was part of her inability to figure out the environments of which she had been a part. She had spoken of not being able to quickly tune in to what was happening around her. One day, I began to sneeze in response to her perfume. She apologized and said it was new. I apologized for my sensitive nasal mucosa. Periodically, during these sessions, which were focused on her despair, anxiety, guilt, and disappointments with her family, I found myself thinking

about her beauty and what a sensual experience with her might be like. I thought myself to be unprofessional. She continued to work hard and was making progress in overcoming her phobic tendencies. Many sessions later, she brought me a small gift and in response to my questions, embarrassedly confessed her romantic love for me. In another session, emboldened, she suggested how she longed to comfort me the way only a woman can. I felt an immediate charge of arousal. Her brief foray into seduction helped me to see that I had missed the point earlier. I was not unprofessional. I was blinded by the guilt over my pleasure and could not see that my erotic fantasies were a reflection of hers.

An erotic countertransference can be much more extensive than a brief fantasy during a session. It is not the ardent words that the patient utters at a particular moment but something more basic in his or her character that stimulates the therapist's intense reactions. On a rare occasion, the therapist thinks, "This patient is perfect for me!" Although the therapist's memories, associations, dreams, and other subjective responses to the patient may lead to a linkage to other important people in his or her past, this does not eradicate the patient's appeal. It simply provides the therapist with an appreciate of how one fresh and unique person can reactivate memories and conflicts. Such erotic countertransferences are invitations for ongoing dialogue within the therapist about the past and the quality of his or her present life. Often they become a motive for entering therapy or using an already existing therapy to explore the subjective love that has occurred.

His first psychotherapy patient as a 25-year-old graduate student was "incredibly physically attractive" to him. He could not stop thinking about her after their sessions. He did not think that the problems that she sought help for at the student health center were anything more than typical problems of young women at college. Her interest in art, her musicality, and her sense of humor seemed perfect for him. She would have blended in nicely with his family's sensibilities. She, in fact, seemed a big improvement over the woman he recently had broken up with, and after some of their sessions, he felt intensely sad about his love life. He was too embarrassed by these reactions to her to discuss this with his supervisor. Therapy ended with the end of the school term; her school and career anxiety seemed better. Four years later, he was able to share this experience for the first time in a seminar designed to discuss these issues. "I wonder what was really troubling her. I think I may have missed it entirely because I was so self-preoccupied."

KEEPING LOVE THERAPEUTIC

Elements within the therapist and patient protect the therapist–patient dyad from sexual behavior. These elements keep the powerful emotional forces in check so that the honorable goal of improving the patient's capacities to live a healthier psychological life is not jeopardized.

The Cultural Tradition

The long tradition of the therapist as helper stems at least from the days of Hippocrates; societies entrust and expect their physicians to always act in the patient's behalf. This expectation is canonized in the Principles of Medical Ethics, which every mental health professional discipline endorses.[5]

The developmental underpinnings of erotic transference are inevitably incestuous: the authority, responsibility, and understanding of mental life that therapists bring to their professional relationships create a power differential that harkens back to the dependency of children on their parents. There is now a broad cultural awareness that children normally experience a series of intense bodily feelings, sexual ambitions, and fantasies about their parents as they develop from the helplessness of early childhood to independence in late adolescence.

Their Lives Outside of Therapy

The therapist and the patient also have personal lives outside of their therapeutic relationship. When these lives are satisfying, they each have a protection against the erotic pressure of therapy. When both have highly unsatisfactory personal lives, the temptations are greater.

The Patient's Understanding of What Is Proper

Many patients in long-term psychotherapy fully understand that they are both participant and observer in their therapy hour and in their lives outside of therapy. Many also understand that they can allow themselves the open expression of their longings simply because they can trust the therapist not to gratify their sexual longings. This generates a strange paradox: the same person who insists upon gratification of the sexual longing may be terrified that the therapist may actually act on the offer. This leaves the patient disappointed no matter what the therapist does. Time-honored therapeutic tradition insists that the patient be allowed the dignity of being sexually frustrated.

When patients let their therapists know about their love, they expect to be helped to benefit from it. They understand that it is part of the process. Sexually offending therapists often rationalize their sexual behavior with the patient as being for the patient's benefit.[6] In the regression of therapy, patients may request and accede to the therapist's sexual advance. Even as it is occurring, most patients know that it is improper. "I don't care!" fleets through their minds.

WHO HAS EROTIC TRANSFERENCES?

Patients with severe emotional problems, usually referred to as having borderline psychopathology or worse, who were sexually abused are often used as examples to illustrate erotic transferences.[7] Many of these people experience a relatively fast, dramatic, troubling response to the therapist. These women and men illustrate many aspects of the complexity of erotic transference—acting out rather than remembering, willingness to be a sexual partner in return for parental affection and special consideration, and a too-rapid trust of the therapist.

A 36-year-old chronically depressed, overwhelmed mother of teenagers, recently discharged from her job as a teacher because of concentration problems, had an accurate emerging sense that her marriage was falling apart. Shortly thereafter, she suddenly developed a relentless genital excitement. When her arousal problem did not go away with medication adjustments and further discussion, her psychiatrist of several years hypnotized her. She was able to remember for the first time images of being her father's sexual partner at age 6 to 8 years. She was referred then to me.

During the fourth session, I was resting my arm on a nearby empty chair and slapped the top of its back a few times to emphasize the point I was making. A few moments later, she was sitting in the chair with her head on my shoulder. I was shocked and said, "What *are* you doing?" "You told me to come here, so I came over." "*What?*" "You motioned to me to come sit in the chair next to you. Anyway, I want to be closer to you." "Please *return* to your seat!"

Her genital excitement was the leading edge of her memories of thinking that she was her father's favorite because he chose her as a sexual partner. As her dysphoric life worsened, her genital excitement seemed to be a regressed way of remembering when an important man seemed to love her. As we worked out the details of her abuse, she became briefly psychotic, thinking that there was a little man, a devil, residing in and hanging out of her vagina. Antipsychotic medication and a hospitalization helped her to recover her reality testing and to talk of her guilt and sense of herself as evil. But she continued to be markedly emotionally disabled, despite her progress dealing with her incest. Five years and three therapists later, she continues to be emotionally unwell and described as borderline.

Such dramatic examples are quite misleading. They suggest to the student that only deeply disturbed persons such as those with hysterical or borderline characters have erotic transferences. This is very far from the truth. Ongoing therapy stimulates many private thoughts, feelings, and conflicts in everyone, men and women, regardless of their orientation or the quality of their actual love lives. Eroticism is a normal part of living, attaching, and loving and it is usually manifested in long-term therapy when the therapist is willing and able to see it.

WHAT IS A THERAPIST TO DO?

Of course, therapists can and do instruct their patients about what they consider appropriate behavior within the therapy hour. Some therapists are particularly fearful of patients' loving feelings if they are discussed in erotic or sexual terms. This seems particularly true for women therapists with their heterosexual male patients. Fear of the sexual danger of men does not disappear because one is a therapist. There are daily reminders to all women that some men can easily misperceive a woman's behavior, thinking it to be sexually inviting. A man sexually out of control and a woman subtly sending provocative signals are recognized dangers. Women therapists often have a dread of a man's erotic transference because it is imagined both as a man out of control and a woman who has sent signals.

When a heterosexual man whose love life is seriously deficient is in psychodynamic therapy with a woman, the therapist should expect that he will eroticize their relationship some of the time. The major question is, "Will the two of them be able to discuss the dimensions of this love?"

> A 50-year-old therapist, in practice for 5 years since her late-in-life training, was reporting to colleagues on her individual therapy with a 32-year-old unhappily married man. She seemed a little uncomfortable with his confession that he thought he loved her and was having a lot of thoughts of being with her. She reported that she did not respond beyond continuing to listen. The next session, however, she realized that his "thoughts of being with her" meant that he was having images of lovemaking and intercourse. She became distressed in the conference over this, could not remember what she said to him, but said incredulously to her colleagues, "I'm old, what does he want with me!" She jokingly asked if she could transfer him to another therapist. We tried to help her. This was the first time she could recall a man having sexual thoughts about her in therapy.

Women therapists are sometimes taken aback by the erotic feelings of their women patients. Their surprise is a combination of the ordinary shock that occurs when any therapist discovers such feelings in any patient and from the shock that an apparently heterosexual woman can have homoerotic love. Rather than become preoccupied with whether to think of the woman as heteroerotic, homoerotic, or bierotic, it is prudent to simply listen and try to understand what life experiences are surfacing with this leading edge of transference love.

> A 45-year-old recently widowed woman had begun psychotherapy with a resident while her 20-year-older asexual husband was dying of a rare neurological disease. The doctor had consistently been supportive and able to help her to verbalize much of the pain and fear associated with her husband's illness and death. Three months into therapy, the patient spoke of loving her sessions, then of loving her doctor, remembering everything that she ever

said to her, and then became anxious. In supervision, the doctor and I discussed the possibility that the patient was having sexual feelings toward her. We reviewed how important the relationship had been for both of them since this patient was helping the doctor to realize much about psychotherapy and both have genuinely cared about each other. We wondered whether the patient might worry that her erotic feelings meant that she was a lesbian. In the next session, the patient was skillfully helped to share her erotic dream—"I came into your bed. You looked lovely and calm. I snuggled at your warm breast, rubbing my cheek against your breast and was cuddled by you—very sexy!" She then told the doctor about her sexual abuse, her hatred of men, and her wish that she was homosexual. "I like you, woman to woman, admire you, think about you too much. I've been thinking about you lately, like a crush. I don't think I could have lived through this time without being crazy without you. I don't remember my mother ever comforting me. She was in love with my brothers and always busy with the other children. . . . (Angrily) My father fucks me and nobody knows anything about it! (Cries) No woman ever comforted me."

Their relationship assisted this patient in the reconstruction of her life as a single person. Sexual feelings did not again come up, but their love, respect, and appreciation for one another remained palpable.

After this session, the resident had a new confidence in her ability as a psychotherapist. The idea of a woman patient being in love with her was no longer threatening. Her mastery of this anxiety about being the object of homoerotic imagery and her ability to perceive that the patient's love was real and would lead to the other stories she needed to share helped both of them.

Imagine, however, that the dreamer in this resident's psychotherapy was a man instead. Would it have been as easy to sit calmly while the man described his kissing of her breast? Perhaps, but generally, I think it would have been more difficult. What the therapist already knows of the man, how she understands his patterns and struggles, and the balance of love and aggression that she perceives the imagery to contain will determine how safe from sexual assault and from guilt about being sexually provocative she feels.

Upon hearing descriptions of imagined sexual behaviors, therapists have to decide whether to say nothing, to comment on the closeness that the imagery expresses, to wonder about the aggression inherent in telling it, or to review the rules of abstinence. These decisions must be made on a situation-by-situation basis. If the patient and the therapist are to continue to work productively together, however, they both have to become interested in what the imagery means. There is no reason to think that it means only one thing. The imagery may reflect both love and anger, both a wish to give pleasure and to dominate, to be both a grownup and a child. Saying nothing or reviewing the abstinence rule of therapy often signals to the patient not to bring such affect states up again.

The homosexual man described in Chapter 13, who confessed to wanting to be a girl, developed a sudden resistance in therapy. He came late twice, once getting lost on the way to my office, and came at the wrong hour for his appointment on a third session. When I told him I did not believe this was an accident or an unconscious mistake, he related that he was very bothered by his wish to have sex with me. "Tell me more!" What followed was a fantasy of massaging my feet, caressing my legs, performing fellatio, and holding me in his arms while I slept from my orgasmic pleasure. "What about you? Do I give pleasure to you?" "No, I'm just happy taking care of you." This led us to discussions of his childhood, low self-esteem, his incest with his brother in which he served in this same manner, and sadness that none of his relationships are reciprocal or involve any love. Thereafter, he was on time.

When I was younger, such descriptions of homosexual behavior involving me were much more stressful to me. Now I have more intellectual defenses to understand and deal with them. I view them as an important part of the therapy process, one that adds a great deal to the patients' acceptance and understanding of themselves in all their paradoxical complexity.

BEA—A CASE HISTORY

I met Bea, a woman in her late 30s, during an evaluation of her and her husband in their final attempt to seek help for their unsatisfying marriage. It was apparent that she had no interest or ability to remain married. She appeared to be in need of individual therapy: she was unable to sleep, indecisive about whether to divorce, unable to elaborate on anything that she said, and frequently got derailed in mid-sentence. She literally could not sit still when her husband spoke. "I just cannot listen to his superficial descriptions any longer!" He stated sadly that he only wanted simple things out of life like his wife to be happy to see him, to be home to cook some nights, to be sexually receptive and responsive on occasion, and to be willing to attend some of his professional functions. She was afraid to be alone, pessimistic about living, frightened of the void within her, and felt suicidal. When I said that she was depressed, she replied that she could not distinguish between depression and misery.

I was shocked when she requested that I become her psychotherapist. I felt that I had made little emotional contact with her; she had avoided eye contact most of the time. In the beginning arduous months of weekly therapy, she did not know what she felt or what she was entitled to say. She was demoralized and could find no reason to continue living despite her high level of professionalism in her field. She felt that with the exception of her child, she was unable to love. She claimed never to have had any sexual desire.

Within a year, however, Bea began saying that she was a transformed woman. In terms of her presenting problems, she was correct. The most important of these changes was that she had been able to fall deeply in love for the first time in her life—so passionately that her body spoke to her of desire and arousal in unmistakable fashions. The problem was that I was the object of her love. Bea eventually reported to me that she fell in love with me during our first session. (I was incredulous.)

Bea did not seem to grasp that her childhood and her adulthood bore a relationship to one another. From the beginning, she was loath to discuss her background. The following information emerged grudgingly in bits and pieces. She was the youngest and most talented of three children from a well-to-do family. Bright, winsome, beloved by her parents, extended family, and friends, she recalls always having what she wanted. Her long-suffering mother did not allow the expression of anger and fled to solitude whenever she was sad. During the patient's early years, her mother was frequently alone as she coped with her husband's affair which led him to move to another city when Bea was 6. Although he returned to see "his little girl" and they slept in the same bed without sexual contact on his occasional visits, he died of cancer when she was 9, never having permanently returned to the family. Bea could not acknowledge to herself that he was dead until her senior year in high school. In college, she had a series of crushes on professors, but never had any romantic involvement with peers. Within several years of graduation she married because it was time and her family approved of her loving suitor. She found him awkward and a bit dull. He promised to support her musical career, which blossomed progressively. When Bea tried to tell her mother about her marital unhappiness, she would not listen, feeling both that it was a disgrace on the family and that women had to learn to adjust to such things and value what is positive in life.

Her early therapy dealt with what she was feeling and why it was so hard to share it. She had no anger or sadness in the beginning—only agitation when I perceived these affects to be present. When I wanted to talk about the loss of her father, she either silently stormed or sarcastically derided me for Freudian thinking.

Her frequent aggression toward me always had an ingenuous quality. I knew she was enjoying our relationship immensely because of her pleasurable staring at me during the session, and her long long looks at me when they were over, frequently followed by some pretense to return to ask a question. It took four sessions of uncomfortable silence, angry accusations, and flat denials to acknowledge that she felt a "pleasure in being here and a kind of love for me."

Within several months, my attitude toward her changed. I used to tell myself that I was a veterinarian psychiatrist with her—another difficult silent person. Soon, however, I was enjoying the unpredictability and the camouflages of our relationship. She was quite bright, I was learning about classical music, and she was hungry for the benefits of therapy. What she said to the contrary made me think of the phrase. "She protesteth too much."

We understood that she could not put into words what she experienced through music and that I would not be able to entirely capture her feelings. Still, she and I were pleased at how often I was able to know what she felt, and to help her say it incisively. She would often explode at me, "Why should

I say it, you already know what it is?" or "There is no privacy from you." She listened intensely to me and complained often that I was too quiet in therapy.

I learned to distinguish several of her affect states from her subtly different stares and facial expressions. When I was feeling narcissistically gratified she tended to be thinking how lovely I was. Sometimes, however, she stared in the pleasure of being reunited. At the end of the sessions, I was often annoyed at her one-long-final-look-please stares.

At least once a session for the first year, she managed to describe me as cruel—my silence, my refusal to talk about myself, my not attending her performance, my repetitive focus on the relationship of what she was feeling about me to her past life. Sometimes, these accusations felt like schoolgirl invitations for me to tell her how much I loved her.

She felt that music, not language, was her best form of expression. She was awed by how I put words and ideas together. One day, she gasped at the beauty of my amaryllis (an exceptionally lovely flower) in bloom. The sight of it provoked powerful emotions in her silence. She had not noticed the plant during the 5 weeks it had been growing in the same spot. Although she could not express what was happening in her, I felt that it drew her closer to me because she realized that, like herself, I had some appreciation of aesthetics. The flower was important to her because she had long complained about the poor quality of the pictures I had on my walls and used to wonder about my poor eye. The amaryllis meant that we shared at least some aesthetic sensibilities. From many such experiences, the idea that I was the perfect man for her attained a great intensity.

One day, she wanted a picture of me. "Why?" I asked. "So I can kiss you!" The next session, she brought in a camera. Again, I refused. The next session she brought me a necktie for Christmas, which, after much conflict, I decided not to refuse. The following session, she wore the same tie! During the next six weeks, she spoke of leaving treatment because I was sadistically unwilling to love her back. While walking out of the door during a February session, she asked to delay her next appointment by two days. Without exploring why, I said yes, unaware that she had moved the session to Valentine's Day. When she came bearing presents, I could not contain my annoyance. "I thought I made it clear that I did not wish to receive presents and I told you I would refuse them! Don't you see that you are setting me up to hurt you?" Her face changed to solid pink. She was mortified and speechless. This now desolate woman sat eating the rich chocolates one by one and weeping silently. When she was finished 15 minutes later, she tore Kleenex into small pieces and then broke the expensive pen she had purchased for me into pieces. She was my last patient of the day; when I left the parking garage I could see that a car was parked in the wrong lane in ongoing traffic. As I drove closer, I saw her sitting in it crying. The car was not damaged. I quickly drove around the block, finally having decided to help her out of this dangerous spot. When I returned a minute later, she was gone. She never mentioned the incident.

For the next three months, her sessions focused on her sense of emptiness and her sudden overeating. Rather than stopping her pursuit of me, she intensified it. She was now able to talk directly about loving me and leaving me, knowing herself better, and to my great chagrin, denying that she was in treatment. "I pay you just to see you." She was always offended whenever I mentioned that loving was part of her therapy. "I do not love you in your therapist role; I love you the person!" I wanted to scream at her that she didn't even know me the person, but I knew better—she knew plenty about me just by being with me in therapy. "You are just there, looking lovely, and doing what you are so good at—torturing me!" She complained that the restraints of our relationship were enormously frustrating. "Kiss me, let me touch you. Make love with me." Several times while leaving she angrily pushed against me and then smiled that she found a way to touch me.

Most of the remaining tumultuous sessions were a mixture of two themes: You must find a way to be with me forever; I must, but I cannot leave you. She was in agony. However, she was now a divorced woman living alone without fear, able to sleep, working productively, not suicidal, and eager to live a long life to see how things worked out. She doubted that she could ever love another man, although I repeated that I hoped that she would.

In one of the final sessions Bea uncharacteristically mused, "How did I get better?" A few minutes later she calmly said she thought that she had worked out her Oedipal complex with me. Her final answer, however, was, "I fell in love and stayed in love with you. It was not just transference! You have to remember, Dr. Levine, I thought I couldn't love anybody. And this has been worth everything to me."

SUMMARY

Despite their high frequency and the fact that they have been described in psychiatric literature for almost a century, loving and sexual feelings in therapy have proven a troublesome topic for mental health professionals. Training programs typically do not deal with the subject in any depth. When erotic "transference" is discussed in therapy, the therapist tends to defensively emphasize the historical aspects of the patients' feelings rather than to legitimize the experience of loving the need-fulfilling therapist. Erotic "countertransference" is usually left out of supervision because of a combination of the trainee's embarrassment and the supervisor's respect for privacy—often to the detriment of the therapist's learning. With some supportive assistance, therapists may readily learn how to calmly accept the patient's love, how to deduce the patient's unspoken preoccupations from personal fantasies, how to use the mutual respect to facilitate emotional growth, and how to handle the homoerotic potential in heterosexuals. Although the conceptual lessons are not in themselves difficult, patients' demanding erotic feelings may be burdensome and test the ethical fiber of the therapist.

REFERENCES

1. Person ES: The erotic transference in women and in men: Differences and consequences. *Journal of the American Academy of Psychoanalysis*, 1985; 13:159–180.
2. Blum H: The concept of the eroticized transference. *Journal of the American Psychoanalytic Association*, 1973; 21:61–76.
3. Frayn DH, Silberfeld M: Erotic transferences. *Canadian Journal of Psychiatry*, 1986, 31:323–327.
4. Frayn DH: Intersubjective processes in psychotherapy. *Canadian Journal of Psychiatry*, 1990; 35(5):434–438.
5. American Psychiatric Association: *The Principles of Medical Ethics and Annotations Especially Applicable to Psychiatry*, Washington DC, American Psychiatric Association, 1989.
6. Gabbard GO: *Sexual Exploitation of Patients*. Washington, DC, American Psychiatric Press, 1990.
7. Gabbard GO: *Psychodynamic Psychiatry in Clinical Practice*. pp 437–448, American Psychiatric Press, 1990.

Index